Critical Approaches to Superfoods

Also Available from Bloomsbury:

Making Dinner, Roblyn Rawlins and David Livert
Making Taste Public, edited by Carole Counihan and Susanne Hojlund
Organic Food, Farming and Culture, edited by Janet Chrzan and Jacqueline A. Ricotta

Critical Approaches to Superfoods

Edited by Emma McDonell and Richard Wilk

BLOOMSBURY ACADEMIC
LONDON • NEW YORK • OXFORD • NEW DELHI • SYDNEY

BLOOMSBURY ACADEMIC
Bloomsbury Publishing Plc
50 Bedford Square, London, WC1B 3DP, UK
1385 Broadway, New York, NY 10018, USA
29 Earlsfort Terrace, Dublin 2, Ireland

BLOOMSBURY, BLOOMSBURY ACADEMIC and the Diana logo are trademarks of
Bloomsbury Publishing Plc

First published in Great Britain 2020
This paperback edition published in 2022

Cover design: Charlotte James
Cover image © Claudia Totir / Getty Images

A catalogue record for this book is available from the British Library.

Library of Congress Control Number: 2020945419

ISBN: HB: 978-1-3501-2387-8
          PB: 978-1-3501-9534-9
          ePDF: 978-1-3501-2388-5
          eBook: 978-1-3501-2389-2

Typeset by Integra Software Services Pvt. Ltd.

To find out more about our authors and books visit www.bloomsbury.com and sign up for
our newsletters.

Contents

List of Figures   vii

About the Contributors   viii

Acknowledgments   xi

1   Tracking Superfoods: An Introduction   1
    Emma McDonell and Richard Wilk

Part One   Making Foods Super

2   From Seasonal Specialty to Superfood: Almonds, Overproduction,
    and the Semiotics of the Spatial Fix   17
    Emily Reisman

3   "The New Pomegranate": Rooibos Magic, Traditional Knowledge, and
    the Politics and Possibilities of Superfoods   37
    Sarah Ives

4   Extractionist Logics: The Missing Link Between Functional Foods and
    Superfoods   57
    Christy Spackman

Part Two   Working Miracles

5   "A Really Good Story Behind It": Moringa Bars and Venture Capital
    Funding   79
    Julie Guthman

6   The Miracle Crop as Boundary Object: Quinoa's Rise as a "Neglected
    and Under-Utilized Species"   95
    Emma McDonell

7   What Makes Food Super? The Post-eugenic Promises of Fish Flour
    and Other Super Powders   119
    Hannah LeBlanc

Part Three Superfood Trajectories

8   From Superfood to Staple? Tracing the Complex Commoditization of
     Kale   135
     Marvin Joseph F. Montefrio and Anacorita O. Abasolo
9   The Global Açaí: A Chronicle of Possibilities and Predicaments of an
     Amazonian Superfood   149
     Eduardo S. Brondizio
10   Amaranth's "Rediscovery" in Mexico: A Path Toward Decolonization
     of Food?   169
     Florence Bétrisey and Valérie Boisvert

References   187
Index   216

List of Figures

9.1a   Symbolic values and narratives associated with the açaí palm and
        fruit. Figure by Eduardo Brondizio   151
9.1b   Value aggregation of the pulp produced in 1 hectare of açaí fruit.
        Figure by Eduardo Brondizio   153
9.2   Phases of expansion in transformation and consumption of
        açaí fruit, from a regional staple to a national favorite to an
        international craze. Figure by Eduardo Brondizio   159
9.3   Data from four açaí processors, 2006–7, Ponta de Pedras and
        Belém, Pará State. Figure by Eduardo Brondizio   163

About the Contributors

Anacorita O. Abasolo is currently pursuing her PhD degree in Environmental Science at the University of the Philippines, Los Baños. She specializes in agro-environmental sustainability assessment and her current research is on the impacts of climate change on agri-fishery communities.

Florence Bétrisey holds a PhD in Geography and works as a postdoctoral researcher at the Institute of Geography and Sustainability of the University of Lausanne, Switzerland. She works on the genesis of institutional arrangements in the (agro-)environmental field and the role scientific knowledge plays in these processes. Her current research focuses on crop genetic diversity and on the diversity of instruments designed to preserve and enhance it.

Valérie Boisvert is a Professor of Ecological Economics at the Institute of Geography and Sustainability of the University of Lausanne, Switzerland. Her work focuses on the political economy of biodiversity, the valuation of wild plants and local landraces, and the development of biodiversity-related markets. Her current research concerns agrobiodiversity management in the context of agroecology and alternative agricultures.

Eduardo S. Brondizio is a Distinguished Professor of Anthropology at Indiana University, Bloomington, and directs the Center for the Analysis of Social-Ecological Landscapes. For over thirty years, he has maintained a field-based research program in the Brazilian Amazon focusing on interactions between rural and urban populations, development policies, commodity markets, and climate change, and the governance of the region's increasingly complex mosaic of urban, agricultural, indigenous, and conservation areas. Brondizio served as Co-Chair of the Global Assessment of Biodiversity and Ecosystem Services of the Inter-governmental Science-Policy Platform on Biodiversity and Ecosystem Services.

Julie Guthman is a Professor of Social Sciences at the University of California, Santa Cruz, where she teaches and conducts research on the politics of food and agriculture. Author of three award-winning monographs, an edited collection, and over forty articles in peer-reviewed journals, her research has been supported by the National Science Foundation, the USDA, the John Simon Guggenheim Foundation, the Radcliffe Institute, and the Rockefeller Bellagio Center. Currently she is the principal investigator of the UC-AFTeR Project, a multi-campus collaboration exploring Silicon Valley's recent forays into food and agriculture.

Sarah Ives teaches Anthropology at City College of San Francisco. Her research focuses on environmental studies, gender studies, comparative studies in race and ethnicity, and southern Africa. She published her first book, *Steeped in Heritage: The Racial Politics of South African Rooibos Tea*, in 2017. Her work has appeared in *American Ethnologist, American Anthropologist,* and *Gender, Place and Culture,* among other peer-reviewed journals and popular media.

Hannah LeBlanc is a Mellon Postdoctoral Fellow in the Science and Technology Studies Department and Society for the Humanities at Cornell University. Her research addresses the history of food and nutrition science in the twentieth century, with a focus on US militarism and Cold War culture.

Emma McDonell is Visiting Assistant Professor of Anthropology in the Social, Cultural, and Justice Studies Department at the University of Tennessee, Chattanooga. Her current research explores the cultural politics of quinoa's commercialization and, more broadly, questions of race, power, and coloniality in agricultural commodity chains. She is currently working on a book about the quinoa boom and bust in Peru.

Marvin Joseph F. Montefrio is Assistant Professor of Environmental Studies at Yale-NUS College in Singapore, specializing in critical agrarian and food studies. His current research interest examines the cultural politics and political ecology of food in the context of sustainability and globalization.

Emily Reisman is an Assistant Professor of Environment and Sustainability at the University at Buffalo (SUNY) and holds a PhD from the University of California, Santa Cruz. Her research examines the politics of knowledge in agri-food systems, combining agrarian political economy, agroecology, and feminist science studies.

Christy Spackman is Assistant Professor, jointly appointed between the School for the Future of Innovation in Society and the School of Arts, Media, and

Engineering at Arizona State University. Her work examines the ways that science and technology are used to manage sensorial experiences, and how those managed experiences in turn shape everyday relationships with environments. She is currently working on a book tentatively entitled *Making Nothing*.

Richard Wilk is Distinguished Professor and Provost's Professor Emeritus at Indiana University, and is Director of the Open Anthropology Institute. He has also taught at the University of California (Berkeley and Santa Cruz), New Mexico State University, and has held visiting professorships at University College London, Gothenburg University, the University of Gastronomic Sciences, and Birkbeck College. He has lived and worked in Belize for more than forty years, but has recently begun fieldwork in Singapore with a Fulbright teaching and research Fellowship. Trained as an economic and ecological anthropologist, his research has covered many different aspects of global consumer culture. Much of his recent work has turned toward the global history of food and the prospects for sustainable consumption as a means to minimize climate change. His most recent books are a textbook on the anthropology of everyday life, co-authored with Orvar Lofgren and Billy Ehn, a co-edited collection with Candice Lowe Swift, *Teaching Food and Culture*, and *Seafood: Ocean to Plate*, co-authored with Shingo Hamada.

Acknowledgments

This book was originally conceived at the Critical Approaches to Superfoods Workshop, which took place at Indiana University in 2019. This event, and this book, could not have come to fruition without the generous financial support of the Association for the Study of Food and Society, the Indiana University Bicentennial, the Indiana University College Arts and Humanities Institute, and the Indiana University Department of Anthropology. We thank Sarah Osterhoudt for helping to plan and carry out the workshop, along with the Ostrom Workshop for providing space for the event. And we would like to express our gratitude to the workshop participants whose papers did not make it into the book but shaped the contours of the conversation and helped us define the debates this book outlines.

Tracking Superfoods: An Introduction

Emma McDonell and Richard Wilk

At the turn of the twenty-first century, the "superfood" label took off in US and European retail markets. Once unfamiliar foods like quinoa, turmeric, and açaí suddenly burst onto supermarket shelves and restaurant menus. Even familiar products like cranberries, almonds, and ginger were reimagined as superfoods, suggesting that they have exceptional nutritional powers and curative properties.

The numbers tracking superfoods[1] are impressive. Between 2011 and 2015, global food and drink product launches using the terms "superfood," "superfruit," or "supergrain" increased by 202 percent. In 2015 alone, new superfood launches increased by 36 percent (Mintel Press Team 2016). The market has been projected to double from $19.1 billion in 2017 to $40 billion in 2022 (Technavio 2020). Booming demand for superfoods has even led some countries to reorient their export strategies. Peru's Ministry of Exterior Commerce, for instance, launched the "Superfoods Peru" campaign in 2017 in an effort to attract investment in Peru's agricultural exports by marketing the country as the "land of superfoods" at food product expos around the world. While the rise of the superfood in consumer markets was initially concentrated in the United States, it now extends across the world. According to industry studies, while North America is largest market for superfoods, the Asia Pacific region is the fastest growing (Technavio 2020; see Montefrio, this volume).

Existing academic work tends to depict superfoods as a sham or fabrication—merely a marketing device that fools consumers into spending money on products based on unproven claims. Curll et al. (2016) see superfoods as a case of "food fraud." Many news items in recent years have framed superfoods as ineffective at best and swindles at worst.[2] Consumers here are imagined as dupes, susceptible to unproven claims and lofty promises. The proliferation of superfoods can also be taken as a symptom of weak government regulation and the neoliberal abrogation of public safety in favor of profit-seeking corporations and individual choice.

In this book, we shift focus away from the question of efficacy to ask about what kinds of work superfoods do in the world, and how they acquire, increase, and lose power. Whether or not a food truly cures bodily ailments or unlocks untapped stores of energy, the story of the superfood and popular belief in them have important and dramatic effects on society, politics, and the economy. The chapters collectively move beyond the false binary of real or imagined, fraud or miracle, to better understand the forces that drive superfoods in and out of the marketplace, and the consequences of superfoods for both producers and consumers.

But what exactly is a superfood? As a number of scholars emphasize, the superfood is a marketing strategy used to introduce new products to consumer markets like açaí and quinoa and to rebrand familiar products like almonds and cranberries, giving them new value. More than just a marketing device, the superfood is also a folk category people use to classify foods, revealing their conceptions of the relationship between food and bodies. Some superfoods are imagined as working wonders on the individual body while others are believed to work miracles on the social body (or both) (see chapters by Guthman, LeBlanc, and McDonell). Some superfoods derive their power from supernatural authority or connections to distant Others (see chapter by Bétrisey and Boisvert), and many gain legitimacy from nutritional science (see chapters by Ives and Spackman). Other superfoods are curative, acting as tonics to give extra strength, immunity, or energy to fully functional bodies (see Reisman, this volume).

Some scholars have defined superfoods around their "wholeness," their minimal processing, and "natural" nutritional richness (Loyer 2016a). Yet we increasingly see superfoods in processed, extracted, dried, and powdered forms (see LeBlanc, this volume), transformed into food additives or "shots." In the case of açaí, the farther astray from its "natural" or "whole" form, the more symbolic power it conjures (see Brondizio, this volume). The creation of açaí extract allowed its expansion in global markets, as it entered a dizzying array of energy drinks, energy shots, power bars, bowls, and supplemental powders. Some things maintain a dual quality depending on the context, like ginseng, which is a soothing tea in Europe, but a super-powered medicine in Korea. Similarly, matcha green tea is an essential part of highly ritualized Japanese tea ceremonies while it entered US markets as a superfood now found in lattes and health cookies (Dreher 2018). Superfoods can break out of the boundaries of food entirely, like quinoa shampoo, while still drawing their power from their superfood source.

Most superfoods have powers far beyond those of common staples and everyday foodstuffs. These qualities are often *magical* in the sense that they depend upon metaphor, the supernatural, and well-established principles of sympathetic and contagious magic, common tools in marketing foods and drinks (Wilk 2012). The magical power of superfoods often derives from their origins and putative producers (a kind of contagious magic), from their shape or appearance (e.g., sea cucumber and ginseng), or through the powerful agency of intermediaries (brands like Natura and Goop, and technologies that denature, purify, and symbolically construct these products).[3]

Another way to understand superfoods' power is through the kind of structuralism associated with Mary Douglas and Edmund Leach. Structuralism calls attention to the way that culture is fundamentally patterned by categories, taxonomies, and important boundaries. Douglas argues that certain animals are often taboo if they do not fit into cultural taxonomies of animals, for example, fish that have no scales like catfish. Structuralism draws attention to the power of liminal, ambiguous, and boundary-crossing substances, for example, hair, fingernails, and feces, which are products of the living human body but are not themselves alive. Many superfoods lie on the boundary between nature and culture, food and medicine (Loyer 2016b), or in the case of the probiotics, between the visible and invisible. But deployed in this way, structuralism rarely includes a mechanism for change, a way to understand how and why structures change.

A more dynamic approach to structural boundaries is Star's concept of the "boundary object," something that does not fit into established cultural, legal, and bureaucratic categories, and therefore poses a problem which becomes more and more obtrusive and difficult over time (Star 2010). She argues that eventually the anomalous position of the boundary object leads to a reevaluation and reshuffling of categories, which in turn create new boundary objects since no system can accommodate the many new objects produced by science, technologies, and human creativity. This bears more than a passing similarity to Latour's idea about the "proliferation of hybrids," which follows modern attempts to impose order on the social world: a situation of gradually increasing dissonance which eventually erodes the power of authority and creates opportunities for change (Latour 1993).

The conceptual category of the superfood can also be understood with the tools from cognitive linguistics (see Lakoff 1996; Lakoff and Johnson 1980). While classic theories of language envision a world of discrete platonic categories, cognitive linguists argue that cognitive and linguistic categories are fuzzy, without clear boundaries or common shared qualities. Instead they generally have a "prototype" at their center, and around the prototype a set of categories and objects that belong to the set by virtue of one or more characteristics they share with the prototype. The members of the set are bound together by this relationship to the prototype, not by their relationship to each other. Therefore, many things that otherwise appear unrelated can belong in the same category. Açaí and Soylent share no qualities except edibility, but they can both belong in the category of superfood because they have different relationships with a prototypical superfood. Açaí is exotic, expensive, and flavorful, while Soylent is high-tech, offers complete nutrition, has no particular source, and offers environmental benefits. They have little in common, but both share qualities with prototypical superfoods. In addition, different groups and individuals have different prototype superfoods in mind, which account for the vagueness and semantic flexibility of the term in popular practice, a quality exploited by marketers.

While we initially set out to provide a concise definition of the superfood in this introduction, we soon found the superfood to be a moving target. Every definition we came up with seemed to leave out something that people considered a superfood. Defining them around wholeness excluded the açaí extracts that now dominate açaí consumption outside the Amazon (see Brondizio, this volume). Defining them around their reference to "traditional peoples" and distant Others left out the ways the almond industry has worked to reimagine the familiar nut as the most recent material-semiotic fixes to familiar crises in the almond industry (see Reisman, this volume). Thinking about the superfood in relation to upscale consumer markets omits the ways superfoods are often imagined to work miracles beyond the individual body, as is the case in the miracle foods present in the international development and (increasingly) tech sectors.

Thinking about superfoods through prototypes offers a more complex understanding of the category itself that demonstrates dynamics of pliability, fuzziness, and change. Rather than thinking about the superfood as a classic concept defined by a set of necessary and sufficient conditions that strictly differentiate between what is inside and what is outside the conceptual boundary, thinking with prototypes helps us understand how so many diverse products have come to be imagined as superfoods that appear to have little in common: yogurt, bee pollen, chocolate, Soylent, and blended superfood powders.

Superfoods and Their Relatives

We consider functional foods, probiotic foods, drug foods, and supplements as allied categories to the superfood, all occupying the fecund space between food and medicine, and overlapping significantly with superfoods in ways that blur boundaries. The term "functional foods" was first invented in Japan to describe products that could help prevent lifestyle-related diseases, and entered US parlance during the deregulatory era that Spackman (this volume) describes. Often considered synonymous with nutraceuticals (a portmanteau of nutritional and pharmaceutical), the term "functional food" is generally used to refer to food products fortified with vitamins, minerals, or other substances through what Spackman calls "the technological wizardry of industrial food." While products have been fortified since the early twentieth century (e.g., milk enriched with vitamin D, iodized salt), the term usually describes the dizzying array of new products entering markets with unverified and vague health claims like increasing life expectancy, delaying or reversing the aging process, adding male "vitality," and supporting the immune system. As Spackman shows, the uneven regulatory landscape of the United States, where health claims did not need corroboration, enabled the rise of the functional food paradigm in the United States.

The shift from the functional food to the superfood paradigm is in part a symbolic one: from referencing individual molecules to highlighting "wholeness." Many of the very same products, once marketed for the specific molecules they contain, were reimagined based on their origins in "whole" foods. As "processed food" became increasingly demonized, the functional food gave way to the superfood, a framing referencing the whole superfood even in the context of a highly processed beverage. At the same time, the rise of the superfood marked a shift in consumer preferences for natural, sustainable, and whole foods that possess powers greater than a sum of their parts.

Dietary supplements are another form of functional food. They are yet another category in the liminal zone between food and medicine, and they often overlap with the super and the functional. Supplements are those things added to "complete" or "enhance" one's diet. They are often ingested in pill or powdered forms, and while they are complementary to foods, they are not themselves food in that they have no flavor or even a bad taste, and they are meant to fill in nutritional gaps in the diet (see LeBlanc, this volume, on the role of invisibility and palatability in powders). The advent of products like gummi multivitamins and chocolate-flavored chewable calcium supplements in the late 1990s again makes the boundaries of the supplement fuzzy. While daily multivitamins began as remedies for insufficient diets, supplements increasingly promise to optimize and enhance one's body. Nichter and Thompson analyze supplements as part of broader "self-projects," saying that "supplement use is part of a larger self-governance project, in which responsible citizens are attentive to changes in the relative state of their health, carefully monitor such changes, and express concern through health related practices" (2006, 180).[4] Rose argues that in the late twentieth century, "the very idea of health was re-figured—the will to health would not merely seek the avoidance of sickness or premature death, but would encode an optimization of one's corporeality to embrace a kind of overall 'well-being'" (2001, 17). Increasingly, supplement stores and aisles include products marketed as "superfood supplements"—highly processed powders or pills with reference to an original superfood, or merely the shadowy category of superfoods.

Herbs and spices with strong flavors are particularly common superfoods, as are those that fit into Mintz's (1985) category of "drug foods" which have physiological effects, such as hallucinogens, stimulants, and soporifics. Many of our contemporary drug foods like tea, coffee, sugar, and cacao became popular among Europeans because of their putative medicinal superpowers, before being slowly absorbed into everyday life (Walvin 1997). Cannabis is a good example of the process of moving from a powerful drug to a common drug food. The relatively recent emergence of "energy drinks" is an interesting case, often blending caffeine with extracts like taurine and guaranine and making reference to superfoods like açaí and guarana (e.g., Sambazon and Guayaki brand yerba mate energy drinks; see Dohrenwend 2019 on the rise of yerba mate).

In recent years, increased scientific and popular interest in gut microbiota has led to the explosion of foods marketed as "probiotic." As American consumers are now paying attention to their gut landscapes, seemingly mundane items like sauerkraut, yogurt, and sourdough bread have taken on exceptional power and have earned shelf space. Meanwhile, kombucha—a once-obscure drink mostly known in the HIV/AIDS community—has become available in gas stations across the United States while kimchi enters the American lexicon. Cultivating "good gut bacteria" can require probiotic shots and pills, falling more within the realm of supplements than fermented foods. There is lively contestation about the authenticity and efficacy of some of these products. The meaning of a "healthy gut microbiota" is vague and complex. The scientific evidence is weak, and easily blends with marketing pitches and diet fads that make a host of claims about how a good gut microbiota can encourage running the gamut to include weight loss, clear skin, energy, regular digestion, and better mental health.

Becoming Miraculous

Miracle foods and miracle crops are a special category of superfood, which are supposed to act on undernourished bodies and societies rather than enhancing well-nourished ones. They are almost always seen as solving larger development dilemmas while they increase food security and cure malnutrition, a dynamic analyzed in the following chapters by Bétrisey and Boisvert, Guthman, McDonell, and LeBlanc. In the curative metaphor they invoke, miracle crops depoliticize highly political problems like poverty and obscuring questions about why people are malnourished in the first place (Ferguson 1990; Kimura 2013; McDonell 2015). LeBlanc's chapter shows that development experts in Chile thought fish flour could work miracles on the social body—in contrast to the highly individualized consumer superfood powders sold in health food markets in the United States. Quinoa is imagined as a potential solution to a host of development problems at different scales: malnutrition in the Andes, global famine relief, poverty, and adaptation to climate change. The contradictions between these problem-solution narratives are obscured when diverse development experts agree upon the "unrealized potential" of quinoa. Guthman's concept of "solutionism" clearly applies to miracle food stories. The fetishized solution (the miracle food or crop) usually precedes the search for a problem to which it can be applied. This backward logic has been common in the international development community for quite some time (see chapters by LeBlanc and McDonell). Now it is being magnified in Silicon Valley pitch nights and crowd-funded projects where the tech sector has begun to apply their "disruption" logic to the problems they see in global food and agriculture (see Guthman, this volume).

Like super foods, miracle foods have fashion cycles. Every few years the international development community rallies around a particular miracle food or miracle crop: high-lysine corn, Golden Rice, orange-fleshed sweet potatoes (Rao and Huggins 2017), fish flour (see LeBlanc, this volume), and moringa (see Guthman, this volume). In the same way charismatic nutrients gain attention only to fade into the background, the associated foods and crops containing the charismatic nutrient go in and out of fashion (Kimura 2013). Much of the rise of a particular miracle food depends upon the ability of coalitions of institutional actors to construct development potential, a dynamic analyzed by McDonell (this volume).

Some products are even miracle crops in the production context and superfoods in the marketing and consumption contexts. Development agencies see value in quinoa's agronomic hardiness in marginal environments, its nutritional content, and its purported ability to alleviate poverty among farmers. At the same time, it is a consumer superfood sold in supermarkets and incorporated in processed foods around the world. Moringa is a similar product, now in its second boom as a miracle crop. In the late twentieth century, it was supposed to remedy deforestation and provide fodder for animals. In its second coming, it is powerful because of its projected allure to wealthy consumers in superfood bars and as a protein shot, and because its sale could purportedly solve poverty and gender asymmetries in the producing communities (see Guthman, this volume).

Along with these overlapping categories, we can also understand how superfoods work through their alter egos, the marginal members of the food category. Falk (1994) argues that the scale from delicious to disgusting is actually a circle that brings foods that are loved into close proximity with those that are shunned. Falk says that this is why it is easy to move from one extreme to the other, suggesting that the avant-garde and marketers are often looking for a particular kind of disgust for the next fashion trend (Falk 1994). In this way, superfoods are a mirrored reflection of what we might call "underfoods," proto-foods, famine foods, and foods eaten surreptitiously because of the fear of shaming.[5] Penny Van Esterik (2006) shows how an algae considered a starvation food in Laos, only fit for human consumption in the most desperate of times, is reimagined as a superfood among wealthy consumers in the United States, driving up its price so it is no longer a practical option in Laos.[6]

Other examples of "underfoods" might be non-nutritive additives like magical frankincense added to food in medieval Europe to counteract poison, crushing pearls into wine, or floating gold leaf in sweet liqueur for visual appeal. Underfoods might include substances like kaolin, often consumed by children but rejected by adults, and adulterants consumed unawares such as sawdust in bread or chalk in milk. We can also think of these substances as negative food additives, food meant only for display like cows made of butter (Rath 2010), or even insults like waiters spitting in food before serving.

Superfoods in Motion

Thinking with prototypes and boundary objects underscores the temporal dimensions of superfoods—the label itself suggests a kind of motion in time, of revival and a better future. Superfoods derive much of their power from their novelty, which is why we see a constant influx of new superfoods to supermarket shelves every year. A 2019 market research study of the global superfoods market suggested: "One of the key trends for this market will be the emergence of new varieties" (Technavio 2020). Instead of reading this trend in terms of simple efflorescence, a constant generation of new markets for superfoods, we see fashion cycles and alternative trajectories.

Because superfoods are constantly in motion, they are also inherently unstable; they cannot be eternally "new." If they do not have powerful companies behind them and close associations with powerful elites, they cannot linger like established luxury brands. They tend to fade if they are not embedded in a cuisine or elevated by a status system like rare delicacies (for example, caviar and truffles). While superfoods can have tremendous symbolic power, over time their very success and growth in popularity tend to lower their status and make them more mundane and commonplace.

This transition can be devastating to existing markets because of the boom-and-bust cycles inherent to market capitalism (Henshall 2012). Initially, superfoods command a high price because of their scarcity, poor market channels, difficulty in transportation, and sometimes high transaction and processing costs. If indigenous or impoverished people depend on this product for part of their subsistence, as is the case with many superfoods, these initial high prices can lead them to sell part of their diet and switch to cheaper foods, with poor consequences for health. Alternatively, in the quinoa case, the price spike led poor urban people (rarely the farmers) to shift their diet toward staples with poor nutrient value, like instant noodles (McDonell 2016). The same high prices draw new actors into the marketplace, build new market channels, in turn lowering transportation, production, and transaction costs. With more "efficient" markets, the producers who initially benefited may no longer be able to compete. As production increases and the market expands, superfoods become cheaper and can then be embedded in routines, new dishes, menus, and everyday life (see Brondizio, this volume). New products normalize superfoods, like quinoa chips, quinoa vodka, quinoa "snack drinks," Cheerios with quinoa ("Ancient Grains Cheerios"), and the fast-food MacQuinoa (sold in Germany).

According to the superfood industry, "quinoa is slowly becoming a mainstream product" (Nyland 2016). When prices come down and profits diminish, agile marketers and fashionable trendsetters start to look for new candidates.

At its peak of popularity there are three possible futures for a superfood beyond a slow decline. Some will disappear entirely and be forgotten, some will acquire new and added qualities that maintain their popularity, while others enter a kind of hibernation with a small or circumscribed group of consumers. The "Royal Jelly" produced by bees to feed their progeny had a spell as a superfood in the 1960s and 1970s, and now it may be on the way back. Yogurt is a good example of a superfood that became entirely mundane and lost much of its power but is now being revived by the trend toward probiotics. Coffee has acquired added features and qualities which have renewed its power. These include new methods of brewing; organic and shade-grown environmental qualities; the philanthropic powers of fair trade, local roasting, and micro-sourcing; adding ingredients like butter for the energy-rich "bulletproof coffee"; and even special qualities acquired by passing through the digestive system of exotic animals. Spirulina is a good example of a superfood that hibernated for many years. It was popular in the 1960s, drawing some of its power from its putative origins among the Aztecs, and it was also marketed as a very early example of an alternative sustainable or "green" product because of its high nutrient value, productivity, and easy propagation. Recently spirulina has seen a revival, bolstered now by its power as an antioxidant.

We should note that there are hundreds, perhaps thousands, of aspiring superfoods, each with a constituency of fans, scientific studies published in obscure journals, producers and agents seeking an audience. Many come from the industry devoted to marginal food supplements and pseudo-medicines touted in endless advertisements on radio and the internet. There are journals and entire consulting businesses devoted to relatively unknown functional foods and additives, and they vie for attention at industry conventions, conferences, showcases, and expos. The proliferation of wannabe and failed super foods, and their difficulty in finding a market are partially a product of the extraordinary degree of competition among health-related products of all kinds, especially in countries with relatively unregulated markets like the United States.

We can identify a few common attributes of those superfoods that succeed in finding a market. Mintz (1985) has proposed that new products are much more likely to be adopted if they fall into a familiar category or role in an existing cuisine and diet. Quinoa worked because it can substitute for rice, buckwheat, or couscous in familiar recipes. The blender and the rise of the "smoothie" have proven a powerful instrument in the incorporation of diverse superfoods that otherwise have an objectionable appearance, taste, or texture. Superfoods can also enter existing dishes in the form of powders (see LeBlanc, this volume), concentrates, or frozen purée. This transformation allows for products that are unwieldy, fragile, or liable to spoil in their fresh or unprocessed forms, like açaí.

Superfoods and the Other

Superfoods derive their power not only from novelty, but also through their connection to non-Western Others. Underlying this emphasis on superfoods' links to non-Western "traditional ways" is an implicit critique of the industrial food system and existing nutritional authority. Marketing products like chia, quinoa, green tea, goji berries, amaranth, açaí, and turmeric regularly invokes connections to living or "ancient" Others, a dynamic Loyer and Knight (2018) call "nutritional primitivism." Indeed, many of our contemporary drug foods like tea, coffee, and cocoa became popular among Europeans because of their connections to exotic lands and peoples, before being absorbed into everyday life and slowly losing their associations with Others. Rather than other cultures, some super foods draw their power from an exotic landscape. Jojoba was a miracle oil in the 1980s, which promised to give America energy independence in its role as a biofuel grown on desert wasteland, while it also had curative and nutritive powers.

The constant demand for novel superfoods connected to marginalized peoples generates what we might call nutritional bioprospecting, the pursuit of "new" superfoods. This bioprospecting brings up familiar dynamics of colonial extractive geographies: many superfoods are dietary staples in the Global South before they became superfoods and are often appropriated from poor and marginal people who rarely benefit in the long run (Finnis 2012). Exotic people lend their power as mysterious and "natural" exotic sources but get little in return. Likewise, early patent medicines commonly started out in the Global South as exotic powerful ingredients, but were then brought to the Metropole to be domesticated, distilled, fermented, measured, graded, and sorted, then mixed together and put in a "modern" container, either for domestic consumption, or then shipped back to the very Global South where they started off as raw ingredients (Wilk 2008). Montefrio and Abasolo's chapter (this volume) on the commoditization of kale in the Philippines reveals a related dynamic: kale was brought to the Philippines by cosmopolitan consumers who had encountered it abroad, and it is now balanced uncomfortably between humble backyard crop and trendy superfood.

Spackman (this volume) traces this extractionist logics operating at multiple scales in superfoods. Seeing nature as a storehouse of untapped molecules underpins the nutritional bioprospecting at play in the pursuit of new superfoods. Nutritional bioprospecting in turn relies upon the development of new technological instruments, such as the ORAC (Oxygen Radical Absorbance Capacity) test, to understand nature at a molecular level and to extract active molecules. The rise of the "molecular imagination" and its associated technological and institutional apparatuses was a necessary precursor to the rise of this particular category of superfood.

This uneven geography brings to the fore questions of intellectual property, dynamics Ives (this volume) traces in the context of rooibos tea.[7] Ives finds that rooibos marketing is currently in flux, transitioning from an emphasis on the tea's rootedness in place and production by traditional peoples to a focus on antioxidant content, reframing rooibos as a nutritional superfood. This shift in emphasis, from knowing the place of production to knowing the body, sets in motion a new set of debates in the politics of heritage, and brings competing scientific and traditional knowledge claims to the fore.

This example also shows that while many superfoods derive their power from connections to "ancient empires" or traditional people, the authority of nutrition science remains privileged. The authenticity of superfoods is always in question, and real or imagined science, including the work of anthropologists, is often used as a certifying authority.

Conclusions

Beliefs in the exceptional curative powers of particular foods are by no means unique to this historical moment or to wealthy health-conscious consumers. While the recent boom in products marketed as superfoods may be unique in its global extent and economic significance, beliefs in the miraculous power of particular foods are common in records of the past. To return to the introduction to this chapter, the authors of this volume understand superfoods in this expansive sense, as foods or crops that people imagine as having unusual capacities to enact change on the individual or social body. Superfoods do not exist a priori; they require creative and inventive acts. They flourish in market-driven consumer cultures, which constantly seek novelty and where progress requires a continuing turnover of products, many of which are designed to have short lifecycles, what Nader (1965) famously called "planned obsolescence." In a sense, the eventual decline of superfoods is baked into the category.

But what about the fate of the notion of a superfood itself? The category of the superfood is a relatively recent invention, and the history of the consumer marketplace shows that categories themselves can lose their power over time. Overuse can eventually lead to "category fatigue," leaving a vestigial term that is basically empty of meaning even though it might still be used on packaging or in marketing. This has been the fate of terms like "natural" and "fresh" in the modern food marketplace, where they are often applied to highly processed and manufactured foods, and items that have sat in cold storage for months or even years. Perhaps, the title of this book will eventually become a historical curiosity, another academic fad that has lost its luster. Instead, we think that the cultural processes and dynamics discussed in these chapters have much broader applicability to understanding how foodways and diet change over time, still a relatively unexplored topic.

Notes

1   Although the word was invented by the United Fruit Company at the beginning of the twentieth century to sell bananas, its power in the consumer imagination has exploded since the beginning of the twenty-first century (UC Davis 2018).

2   Some representative headlines include: "Experts Say Superfoods May Be a Super Scam," "Are Quinoa, Chia Seeds, and Other 'Superfoods' a Scam?" "Superfoods Are a Marketing Ploy," "Are Superfoods Really Good for You or Just Marketing Hype?" (Benedictus 2016; Hancock et al. 2007; Levy 2014; Nestle 2018a; Philpott 2013; Turner 2015).

3   Intermediaries and brands also symbolically rework products depending on their desired audiences. Gwyneth Paltrow's Goop brand and the right-wing radio host, Alex Jones, sell the same products in their online stores, but market it in very different ways (Sonnad 2017).

4   For more the historical development of this dynamic in the United States, see Jackson Lears (1983), who traces the origin of therapeutic culture in the United States back to the late nineteenth century.

5   Examples include possum and skunk in Belize and armadillos in Texas. We might even count some "junk foods" in the United States that are considered shameful by upper-class consumers in particular. Chef David Chang's momofuku restaurants, for instance, worked to turn these "junk foods" like "funfetti" cake mix and

sweetened cereal into expensive and desirable objects of distinction specifically for consumption in social settings.

6   For more on underfoods, see Chera (2020), who invented the term. Finnis's (2012) volume on marginalized foods is also useful for thinking through these processes.

7   For a related study of intellectual property battles over a superfood, see Laura Foster's (2017) book on hoodia, a succulent plant known by generations of Indigenous San peoples that's became part of a booming diet industry in the early 2000s.

Part One

Making Foods Super

From Seasonal Specialty to Superfood: Almonds, Overproduction, and the Semiotics of the Spatial Fix

Emily Reisman

In the twenty-first century, a widening array of fruits, vegetables, seeds, and grains have been crowned "superfoods." Products with superfood status are on the rise, as the market is expected to grow by more than 15 percent annually between 2018 and 2022 (Technavio 2018). Many so-called superfoods carry exotic appeal. Sourced from distant lands and associated with traditional foodways of indigenous peoples, they have been "discovered" through neocolonial encounters (McDonell 2019a; Sikka 2016). The sudden popularity of these products has dramatically reshaped the socioecological dynamics surrounding quinoa in South America (Jacobsen 2011; Kerssen 2015; McDonell 2019a), açaí berry in the Amazon (Brondízio 2008; Weinstein and Moegenburg 2004), argan oil[1] in Morocco (Lybbert et al. 2010; Turner 2014), and baobab fruit in Southern Africa (Wynberg et al. 2015), with many more cases yet to be explored.

Other purported superfoods, however, are neither new nor exotic for American audiences. They are familiar, domestically grown (when in season), fruits and vegetables gaining unprecedented acclaim: almonds, blueberries, broccoli, cranberries, Brussels sprouts, spinach, carrots, avocado, apple, beetroot, and more. Why have such unassuming items in the produce aisle suddenly become heralded as superfoods? What kind of subjectivity does this new superfood framing cultivate among eaters?

As I will show, almonds have risen to superfood status through consistent efforts by almond producer groups to alleviate the pains of chronic overproduction. Rising production from increased acreage and agricultural intensification prompted the Almond Board of California (ABC) to begin funding nutrition science, influencing health-claim labeling, and advertising almonds as a healthy food during the 1990s. The spectacular success of these efforts, as well as concurrent trends toward high protein diets and increased snacking, sent American almond consumption soaring. Such popularity, combined with high-yielding orchard management, supercharged growers' profits and attracted new kinds of investment capital. A resulting planting frenzy promises to boost production by 30 percent in just four years (Fleischmann and Muir 2018), threatening a price crash. While almond marketers go to great lengths to expand their markets geographically and increase sales around the world, the American market requires a shift in strategy to boost buying. As the health message no longer suffices to grow sales, advertisers have shifted registers from wholesome sustenance to superfood spectacle.

Understanding the political economic context of the almond's ascent not only reveals the historical foundation of superfoods as a contested contemporary food phenomenon, but, perhaps more significantly, sheds light on the metamorphoses of food meanings fundamental to agrarian capitalism. To analyze how and why almonds have become a superfood, I draw on historical archives, advertising materials, interviews with current or recently retired almond industry marketing professionals, and observation at the annual industry conference taking place in 2015, 2016, and 2018. First, I root my analysis by arguing for the importance of semiotics to the spatial fix, contextualizing the superfood phenomenon, and grounding my analysis in critical nutrition scholarship. Then I delve into the almond case, charting the ascent of the almond in American culinary culture as a series of material-semiotic fixes to familiar crises of agrarian capitalism. Finally, I use the case of almonds to consider the broader superfood trend and its imagined "super" subjects as produced through the political economy of American agriculture.

Engaging the Semiotics of the Spatial Fix

The structure of capitalist economies incentivizes excessive production, which ultimately drives down prices and profits. David Harvey coined the term "spatial fix" to describe how capitalist economies cope with repeated crises of surplus production through expansion (1981). The perpetual growth of the almond industry both domestically and abroad exemplifies the familiar pattern of a spatial fix to capitalism's internal crises. Harvey's theorization of the spatial fix makes two significant claims: (1) that the instability of overproduction provokes geographic restructuring and (2) that this restructuring is always in tension with the place-bound quality of infrastructures necessary for the production and circulation of capital.

Capitalist economies suffer from cyclical episodes of surplus accumulation which then pose a risk of rapid devaluation. To avoid a painful devaluation period, the ever-unstable accumulation of surplus capital buys itself time through market expansion (Harvey 2006). The drive to expand markets as a spatial fix to overproduction is characteristic of imperialism and the uneven development of globalization (Jessop 2006; Smith 2008). Importantly, the spatial fix is imagined as a solution but functions more like the fleeting "fix" of an addiction, as the problem soon returns (Harvey 2001). The spatial fix provides short-term relief but the underlying predicament is ultimately magnified (Schoenberger 2004).

It is well documented that American agriculture suffers from chronic overproduction (Cochrane 1993; Winders 2009). Where supply management has failed, farm economic viability has depended upon the expansion of foreign markets for American agricultural products (Graddy-Lovelace and Diamond 2017). Expansionism is limited, however, by the purchasing power of those new customers and/or the willingness of the state to subsidize foreign market development. Reallocation of agricultural products to non-food uses, such as biofuels, serves as another strategy, albeit with risks for exacerbating food insecurity (Gillon 2016). While non-food uses might be viable for grains sold for pennies per pound, almonds selling on the commodity market for over thirty times that price can only profitably be sold for human consumption.

Human digestive systems can only physically process so much, making demand for food highly inelastic. In addition, the famed economic principle Engel's Law states that as wealth increases the portion of income spent on food falls (Zimmerman 1932). For these reasons, the food business is supremely competitive. Thus, in addition to off-loading American products abroad and shifting agricultural products toward non-food uses, the body of American consumers itself is increasingly a site of an eternally inadequate spatial fix (Guthman 2015). This is evident in the fact that food marketing over the past few decades has progressively enticed consumers to eat more (Nestle 2013), a pattern of "accumulation by engorgement" (Guthman and DuPuis 2006, 442) with significant public health implications. This spatial fix at the site of the body demonstrates the mutual constitution of production and consumption (Coles 2016), as capitalist processes reshape not only bodily processes but eating practices. The meaning-making processes accompanying such material reorderings merit closer attention.

The spatial fix is a material-semiotic process, with important psychosocial dimensions often downplayed in the historical materialist tradition. It requires a shift in not only the physical spaces a commodity occupies but also the meanings it conveys. Material-semiotics asserts that matter and meaning are fundamentally inseparable (Barad 2007). Scholars using a material-semiotic approach look for the active, ongoing ways in which matter and meaning are co-produced (Law 2019; Mol 1999). In a seminal text insisting on the unity of matter and meaning, Donna Haraway describes bodies as "material-semiotic nodes" that cannot be understood physiologically without their array of accompanying conceptual devices (Haraway 1991, 208). Political economic analyses of capital accumulation often trace commodity flows without attending to the meaning-making practices required for them to function. On the other hand, studies of discourse in the Foucauldian tradition often fail to address how material substances are intertwined with discursive practice. Following Haraway's merging of Marxian attention to the material with post-modern attention to the semiotic (Eglash 2013), I seek to draw political economic and cultural studies of food closer together through a material-semiotic analysis of the relationship between overproduction of a food and its shifting culinary culture. Superfoods, as a distinctly discursive and profoundly political economic phenomenon, provide an illustrative case.

Through the almond case, I find that the semiotics of the spatial fix parallel Harvey's two postulates concerning the material ordering of capitalist economies. (1) The instability of overproduction provokes *semiotic* restructuring; the meanings of almonds must shift to expand their profitable consumption. This fix is the addictive sort which delays, rather than solves, the crisis as meanings (tightly linked with their target markets) can also become saturated.

(2) Meaning-making practices are, like material infrastructure, significant investments which fix the industry to a semiotic configuration from which it is unlikely to deviate without significant cost. Rather than deem this process a distinct "semiotic fix," I wish to highlight the simultaneity of material and semiotic reordering as an inherent, underappreciated, quality of the spatial fix.

Contextualizing Superfoods

There is no agreed upon definition of a superfood beyond a recognition that such a broad claim likely does more to drive sales than to inform eaters ("Superfoods or Superhype?" 2018). The term "superfood," however, has become so widely used that the Oxford English Dictionary began including it in 2007, defining the superfood as "a nutrient-rich food considered to be especially beneficial for health and well-being." As the qualifiers "considered" and "especially" suggest, the superfood concept reflects the belief that a single food can possess an exceptional level of quality for enhancing human wellness. Superfoods are a discourse instead of an actual descriptor of material substance (Loyer 2016b).

The term "superfood" fits within the functional foods category, but with important distinctions. According to nutrition scientists, functional foods are those which "provide health benefits beyond the provision of essential nutrients (e.g. vitamins and minerals) when they are consumed at efficacious levels as part of a varied diet on a regular basis" (Hasler 2002). The framing of functional foods relies on a mechanistic model of the body in which a targeted input can produce a desired result. For example, omega-3 fatty acids are claimed to reduce levels of LDL (Low Density Lipoprotein) cholesterol which in turn reduces risk of heart disease (for more on the history of the functional foods category, see Spackman, this volume).

By contrast, the superfood designation, while rooted in many of the same reductionist claims of nutritionism (Scrinis 2013) and a factory-like conception of metabolism (Landecker 2013), embraces the indeterminate outcomes of a given food. The superfood narrative supplements functionality with an element of enchantment, often suggesting that the benefits of a given food are intangible felt experiences of vitality, high spirits, and the glow of overall wellness (Wolfe 2009). Superfoods claim to stack functions, providing a high density of beneficial dimensions within a single item. They also convey a sense of limitless benefits to consumers, shifting away from the recommended dosage of medically styled discourse of functional foods toward a designation of inherent incalculable goodness. Functional foods call awareness to specific phytochemicals and their benefits, whereas the superfood message is simplicity. Above all, the word "superfood" rolls off the tongue more readily and has gained powerful momentum as a culinary meme.

The superfood phenomenon is part of a broader counter-cultural critique of industrial food systems emphasizing whole foods (in contrast to processed ones) and, to a lesser extent, intergenerational culinary wisdom. Yet it is also a powerful advertising tool eagerly adopted by food marketers. The food industry's use of messaging that critiques industrial food is less a contradiction than the norm (Belasco 2007). Even more importantly, the superfood concept would not be possible without extensive single-food scientific research overwhelmingly, if not exclusively, funded by industry groups (Nestle 2018b). Nutrition scientists are typically much more interested in understanding the impact of diet or specific nutrients on the body than assessing the merits of a single food. Yet for academics relying on external funding for professional advancement, food industry grants are an appealing opportunity to pursue rigorous research that centers on the "compatible interests" of academics and industry (Dixon and Banwell 2004).

While nutrition science cumulatively contributes to the functional food and superfood trends, both terms have raised alarm among nutrition scientists who warn consumers against believing in "magic bullets or panaceas" (Hasler 2002) and emphasize the need for a well-rounded diet (Lunn 2006). The European Union actually banned the use of the word "superfood" on product labels unless accompanied by an authorized health claim in 2007. Thus, superfoods appear to be the latest trend in the corporate co-optation of both the alternative food movement and scientific institutions.

Theorizing Superfood Subjectivities

Eating right has become a powerful "technology of the self" (Foucault 1988) through which individuals govern their own bodies, thoughts, and behaviors. Nutritionism, which considers isolated nutrients as the fundamental unit of food knowledge, is now the dominant paradigm for relating food to wellbeing (Scrinis 2008). The rise of the nutricentric citizen is part of a century-long food system transformation "that has mobilized the material and symbolic values of nutrition with 'a will to govern'" (Dixon 2009).

Critical nutrition scholars point to the ideological projects embedded in American food reform. Early nutrition research emphasized economic efficiency to avoid labor unrest (Biltekoff 2013). The Second World War mobilized nutrition as a tool for instilling service to the nation as a daily routine (ibid.). Mid-century dietary guidelines centered the laboratory as the ultimate site of food expertise in order to control food discourses and forge subjects accepting of state authority over household affairs (Mudry 2009). Alternative food movements emerging in the late twentieth century, knowingly or unknowingly, reinforce neoliberal subjectivities of autonomy, individual responsibility, entrepreneurship, and self-improvement (Biltekoff 2013; Guthman 2008; Türken et al. 2016). Over the last century, food has taken on increasing political weight as a site of perpetual anxiety and a forum for governing our relationship to our bodies (Scrinis 2013).

The burden of food anxieties is distinctly gendered, with food advertising that consistently "holds women responsible for their family's health, status and satisfaction" (Parkin 2007, 11).

Analyses of food reform movements have emphasized the influence of dieticians, nutrition scientists, social workers, and counter-culture entrepreneurs in shaping ideologies of eating—but what about agribusiness? Exposure to advertising has increased with the digital age (Media Dynamics Inc. 2014), and US advertising spending hit an all-time high in 2018 (MAGNA 2018), likely expanding the influence of private sector visions for proper eating. Scholars and popular critics increasingly blame food advertising for undermining food reform efforts by encouraging children to consume fast food, processed foods, and sugary drinks (Bittman 2012; see Boyland et al. 2016 for a meta-analysis of this extensive literature). With the exception of milk (DuPuis 2002) however, little has been said about the social values embedded in promotional campaigns in line with (and at times directly influencing) recommended nutritional guidelines. While agribusiness-funded ads for whole foods might be presumed to reinforce the message of government-issued dietary rules, the controversy surrounding superfoods shows this is not always the case.

Of course, the public and private sectors permeate one another constantly. As political scientists Guardino and Snyder argue, the state is an active participant in the expanded role of corporate promotional media. They define the capitalist advertising and marketing complex as a "range of closely connected corporate and state institutions involved in widening the scope and advancing the power of commercial promotion in the broader economy" (2017). Produce advertising is far less controversial than marketing soda to second graders, but it is no less a pillar of twenty-first-century state-supported agrarian capitalism. While Nestle warns consumers against believing industry-funded nutrition science touting the benefits of blueberries, pomegranates, or pecans (2018b), she does not venture an analysis of how superfood messaging might influence consumers beyond misinforming them. Why has "superfood" status become so central to the produce industry? What kind of work does the superfood phenomenon do for agrarian capitalism? The ascent of the almond provides some clues.

Overcoming the Seasons

Just a century ago, almonds in American culinary culture were a strictly seasonal treat. This dynamic is surprising considering the lack of urgency to consume them directly after harvest, as with perishable fruits and vegetables. It is a reminder, however, that food cultures have historically been closely tied to the temporality of farming. In the Northern Hemisphere, almonds are harvested in late August through October, sold and processed in October and November and, until the mid-twentieth century, marketed exclusively as a winter holiday specialty. Almond cultivation was likely introduced to California by the Spanish missionaries but did not take on a commercial scale until the post-Gold Rush population boom of migrating Anglo-Americans in the 1860s. Orchards gradually took root along the Sacramento River Valley when a growing settler population and a surplus of capital made farming an attractive business opportunity. As word spread of the crop's lucrative potential and orchards expanded, almonds' popularity among farmers began to clash with its culinary niche. There were simply too many almonds to sell them for only a few months out of the year.

Prices were unstable, and growers grumbled they were at the mercy of middlemen who pitted them against one another to keep prices low. The global grain glut of the 1890s prompted a golden age of cooperative organizing in American agriculture (Filley 1929; Saker 1990; Stoll 1998), and almond growers soon followed suit by selling collectively at regional hubs. These regional cooperatives, however, continued to undersell one another. After a painstaking process to overcome mistrust, alliances were forged in 1910 to bring 80 percent of production under the umbrella of a single entity: the California Almond Growers Exchange (CAGE). The influence of this momentous unification cannot be overstated. California affords the only climatic conditions in North America suitable for almond cultivation and growers suddenly had a near monopoly on their product. Cooperation brought astonishing results. In the decade following the formation of the exchange, growers received prices 50 percent higher than before it was established (Tucker 1920, 5).

Good prices set off a planting boom and fears of overproduction were not far behind. In 1919, the crop was double that of 1918. The president of the exchange warned almond growers of a grim future if they failed to address the looming surplus of their product. Because almonds take three to five years to produce their first crop, rapidly expanding young orchards were visible evidence of mounting production on the horizon. Unlike an annual crop, which could be changed year to year in response to market signals, a permanent crop with substantial up-front investment prompted growers to dig in their heels.

"You will have much to worry about … if you fail to supply the necessary funds for advertising and development," he warned (Tucker 1920, 16). The industry faced two challenges: almonds were sold strictly seasonally and were closely associated with special occasions. The exchange found convincing a wholesaler or retailer to stock almonds after January 1 to be "impossible" (ibid., 5). The *American Nut Journal* concluded that to keep up with production, the place of almonds in the American diet must be shifted to "year-round consumption as food" ("The Year's Opportunity" 1920). An early catalog advertisement implored readers to "think of them not as an appetizer merely, or some rare delicacy to be enjoyed at Christmas and then disappear, but rather as an article of food to be kept always in the house" (Cobb Bates & Yerba Co. 1910). Almonds were so tightly linked to the holiday season as to be considered more of a treat, a social activity, or a finishing touch than as a source of nourishment. In retrospect, it is striking that while today almonds are popularly touted as a *superfood*, just a century ago it was novel for Americans to even consider them a food.

Becoming an "Essential Food"

It would not be until the 1960s, after forty years of relentless marketing by the industry, that the seasonal pattern of almond purchasing would transition to year-round buying (Allen 2000, 128). Consumers are not passive recipients of the gastronomic ideals proffered in advertising; culinary conversion takes work. In the meantime, a successful lobbying effort in the 1920s to raise tariffs on imported almonds from Europe gave California growers temporarily relief.

During the Great Depression, when economic collapse drove many to hunger even amid food surpluses, the emerging field of nutrition science took on increasing political import. Under the USDA's (United State Department of Agriculture) expanding role, policymakers sought to educate homemakers in stretching meager budgets through economically efficient nutrition (Atwater 1895). A mechanical view of the body as engine-like simplified food into energetic inputs and outputs, advocating rational calculation over personal satisfaction or cultural significance (Mudry 2009). Eager to be viewed favorably under the influential nutritionist paradigm, the CAGE contracted with a private firm, the California Foods Research Institute, to perform state-of-the-art analyses of the nutritive values of almonds. This institute "worked closely with the exchange's advertising agency, … developed recipes for distribution to news media," and "got the nutrition story to newspapers, radio stations, magazines, cooking schools and scientific publications" as well as to nutrition teachers in rural areas, "dietitians of private and government hospitals, and quartermasters of the Army, Navy and Marines" (Allen 2000, 91). The institute appeared to be laboratory, advertising consultant, and public relations firm all-in-one and was, unsurprisingly, hired by other California commodity groups of the time.

During the Second World War, the US government feared that insufficient nutrition would mean "a slowing down of industrial production [and] a danger to military strength" (Mudry 2009, 61). Armed with quantified nutrition data emphasizing caloric density and energy-building fats, the CAGE successfully lobbied to have almonds designated an "essential food" by the War Manpower Commission (Allen 2000, 93). This meant almond growers received preferential access to gasoline, equipment, and Mexican labor contracted through the Bracero program while other industries were constrained by rations. The spatial fix to overproduction during wartime would not have been possible without enrolling scientific authority to literally redefine the meaning of almonds as "essential" in the eyes of policymakers. The nutritional profile of an almond itself is a material-semiotic object, a characterization of molecules inseparable from their significance for human health. For almond production to materially expand into military rations and the national food supply, it had to successfully morph meaning.

In the post-war era, anxiety over surpluses reemerged as almond production exceeded domestic consumption before the war. In 1945, President Truman reversed a slew of tariffs, which had buoyed American farmers since 1930. Producers feared imports from regions with lower labor costs would flood the market. The industry responded with product differentiation, creating canned and flavored nuts as well as new forms of chopped and slivered nuts to top sweet treats. They secured a purchasing agreement with the USDA school lunch program to buy 5 million pounds of almonds each year. Most significantly, after three years of lobbying in Washington, DC, California growers succeeded in amending the Agricultural Adjustment Act to include almonds and filberts. This meant growers could elect to form a Federal Marketing Order. While originally intended to manage surpluses by restricting sales during bumper crop years and formalizing quality standards, the Marketing Order would eventually become an unprecedented advertising and nutrition research powerhouse.

Scrambling to Sell

As a Federal Marketing Order, the Almond Control Board legally required all almond producers to abide by its standards and to pay a fee per pound for the functioning of the organization. To keep prices from falling, the board could set aside stockpiles of almonds, amounting to as much as 25 percent of the total crop in 1951. The board also created a two-tier pricing structure, selling almonds abroad at half the price of domestic almonds in order to open new markets and off-load the surplus (GAO 1985). But they could not stop growers from planting. Mechanization, increased use of petrochemicals, and technical support from the land-grant universities boosted production per acre as almond acreage continued to expand. Average yields climbed 64 percent between 1949 and 1961. In 1959 the industry faced a crop four times the size of the year prior and launched the "Colossal Almond Crop" promotional campaign. Unlike the war-era focus on nutritional substance, mid-century advertising emphasized almonds as a versatile ingredient for female homemakers and in the expanding market of consumer packaged goods. The success of these efforts attracted even more farmers to convert their land to almond orchards. In 1966, the almond industry and then Governor of California Pat Brown considered acreage limits or removal of immature fruits to reign in surpluses, but citing enforcement challenges, determined new markets were the most feasible option (Allen 2000).

Sales from the exchange doubled between 1960 and 1970. In 1972, almond growers and other commodity groups drowning in surpluses successfully lobbied Congress to amend the marketing order program and allow funds to be used for advertising and market research (GAO 1985). These expenditures had been expressly forbidden under prior legislation. The change was nothing short of revolutionary. By 1981, the board spent 97 percent of its total budget on advertising, promotion, and research and development. Marketing has dominated spending ever since.

The board also incentivized handlers, like the exchange (officially renamed Blue Diamond Growers in 1980), to advertise independently by giving them a credit toward their dues for money spent promoting their own brand. As one marketer explained, "Blue Diamond spent ... because it was kind of free. Because we were getting it back from the Almond Board. So what that did is, you had 20 years of advertising that the size of the business didn't warrant." Government-mandated payments, and incentives for brands to spend, created a flood of promotions.

Just as the first million-dollar almond advertising campaign went public, American purchasing power declined due to oil embargoes and high interest rates. Both Blue Diamond and the Almond Control Board went to work abroad to boost sales, with matching funds from the USDA Foreign Market Development Program. After another decade of making miracles for growers, the

Blue Diamond president lamented in 1979, "virtually every significant potential market in the world is now open to our product … there are no longer the many opportunities for new development that existed some years ago" (Allen 2000, 155). Further compounding growers' woes were Reagan-era economic policies that strengthened the dollar and made almonds more expensive abroad. To maintain and expand markets, almond exporters received government funding through the Targeted Export Incentive Program, which allowed almonds to be sold abroad at below market rates. Over the course of the 1970s, almond acreage doubled again.

Given limited international interest and lower profit margins for products sold abroad, almond growers focused on boosting per capita consumption in the United States. The CAGE president underscored the stark situation, "One doesn't normally ask someone to increase the consumption of a product by more than 40 percent in a single year … but that, in a sense, is what we are being asked to do" (ibid., 158). The cooperative launched an atypically frank television advertisement exemplifying the surplus crisis. Almond growers buried up to their elbows in almonds pleaded with shoppers: *a can a week is all we ask.*

The candid and humorous tone of the ads gave almond growers an unexpected fifteen minutes of fame. The 1980s US Farm Crisis, in which surplus production drove down prices while farmer debt soared, was becoming legible to broader publics at that time through events like the celebrity-sponsored Farm Aid concert of 1985. Almond marketers leveraged the idea of supporting farmers as a civic duty and pursued a spatial fix to their crisis of overproduction through reframing consistent almond purchases as an act of solidarity.

Harnessing the Health Halo

The word "healthy" began popping up in almond advertisements in the 1970s as marketers caught on to emerging trends in "natural" or "whole" foods (Belasco 2007). But it wasn't until the 1990s that the almond industry would begin funding a veritable onslaught of nutrition research to back promotional claims. The motivation was twofold. First, the Food and Drug Administration (FDA) had become increasingly restrictive about health claims made by food advertisers and required scientifically backed justification (see discussion of "regulatory fences," Spackman, this volume). Second, a small group of almond handlers unhappy with the requirement to pay for collective advertising by the Almond Control Board sued, claiming the obligation infringed upon their freedom of speech. They were temporarily successful, and in 1994 brought advertising spending to a screeching halt. The ABC, with an estimated $11.14 million budget in 1995,[2] decided that while waiting for an appeal, they would shift part of their formidable advertising budget into nutrition research. The first order of business was to challenge the low-fat diet craze by showing that almonds contained "good" fats.

"When I first arrived at Almond Board of California in 1999, only two almond nutrition research papers had been published," the board's current Chief Scientific Officer Dr. Karen Lapsley said in 2018. "To date we have [supported] 158 nutrition research peer-reviewed published papers" (Almond Board of California 2018). She estimated in our interview that roughly 75 percent of existing worldwide knowledge about almonds, possibly more, has been supported in some way by the ABC.

Advertisers were particularly keen on finding a recognized icon that would validate their health message. The American Heart Association's (AHA) "heart-check" food certification program provided just such an opportunity, but the AHA held to a strict limit on the fat content of its approved products. Almonds were ineligible. The FDA similarly rejected a proposed statement that nuts reduce the risk of heart disease. After substantial industry efforts, FDA approved a qualified health claim stating, "scientific evidence suggests but does not prove that eating 1.5 ounces per day of most nuts, as part of a diet low in saturated fat and cholesterol, may reduce the risk of heart disease." The almond industry continued arguing their case to the AHA and eventually succeeded in obtaining the heart-check stamp of approval. But it was not easy, and almost certainly never would have happened without ABC's hefty investment.

Health messaging transformed the almond market. The current marketing director of the ABC elucidated how the "health halo" effect has allowed products with almonds as an ingredient to be viewed as healthy by association. "If you think of almonds as healthy and almonds as a great snack, then having an almond as an ingredient in a bar, there's a positive halo that goes to that bar … [it] makes you feel a little better even about eating chocolate, because you're balancing things out." The health halo means any product appears healthier to consumers because it contains an ingredient recognized as healthy. Enthusiasm for the marketing power of the "health halo" is fitting though slightly ironic. The "halo" description was originally a critique of diet foods made by health professionals worried about the tendency for such labels to give consumers permission to binge eat (Chernev 2011; Provencher et al. 2009). Among marketers, the "halo" has lost all hint of disapproval. For driving volume, it's a godsend.

At the ABC, the Nutrition Research subcommittee originally reported directly to the Marketing committee. While the team explored a wide range of topics, "the whole point is to sell more almonds," a senior marketer and longtime Marketing committee member reported:

> It wasn't so direct as the marketing people saying "I want you to work on this, this and that." There was a dialogue. "Well what are you working on that shows some promise for application?" And they'd tell us. And some wise guy like me would say, "Well #1 and #2 actually have commercial application but #3, 4, 5 just stop. It's a waste of time, just don't do it." I mean, there always has to be a certain amount of pure research because you never know what you might learn. I don't want to make it too black and white, but it was marketing driven. Getting back to the mandate of the marketing order itself. It's all about enhancing the value of almonds, expanding markets and basically driving up the price and selling to more people around the world.

As the almond industry set their sights on new international markets, they partnered with nutrition researchers in target countries to root their health claims on foreign soil. They contracted with private nutrition research firms and enticed junior faculty and doctoral students with funding for research investigating almonds' health effects. ABC staff are co-authors on some publications, meaning they have a direct role in study design and analyses of results. For most studies, the board is careful to distance itself from the research process; however, the selection of projects is by design oriented toward perceived sales opportunities. Likewise, researchers prepare proposals to suit the anticipated desires of the ABC.

Unsurprisingly, studies that show little advantage of almonds over other foods drift into relative obscurity while those validating health claims receive top billing in the ABC's nutrition research reports. As veteran food marketers explained, for large consumer packaged goods companies, almonds are too small a portion of their budget to justify a nutrition research investment. More specialized companies lack the funds to pursue such research and are less motivated because the benefits would be spread across the industry. Without the political tool of the marketing order, and the constant threat of oversupply that it simultaneously alleviates and exacerbates, almonds would likely never have been crowned with a "health halo" at all.

Securing Superfood Status

Industry leaders credit the health message with a spectacular growth in domestic consumption. In the 1990s, annual US almond consumption remained relatively stable, averaging 0.63 pounds (0.29 kilos) per capita. By 2017, it reached 2.36 pounds, a rise of 375 percent in less than two decades (USDA 2018). In the early 2000s, phenomenal sales in the United States and abroad, in combination with intensified farming practices, boosted profits for growers. Value per acre averaged $1644 in the 1990s; by 2011 it topped $5000 per acre and peaked in 2014 at an unheard-of $8600 per acre. Lured by attractive returns, California growers converted row crops like cotton and tomatoes to almonds and investors rushed to join the boom. Bearing acreage surged from an average 430,000 acres in the 1990s to over 1,000,000 acres in 2016. An intensifying drought beginning in 2012 drove prices even higher as buyers feared reduced irrigation would produce a short crop. By 2016, the ABC anticipated a 30 percent increase in production within four years. Fearing an oversupply, the board successfully petitioned growers and the USDA to raise the per-pound fee by 33 percent for three years in order to fund additional marketing efforts (7 CFR § 981 2016).

At roughly the same moment, the board shifted its nutrition research program from "health conditions" such as heart disease and diabetes toward "wellness and vitality" (Dreher 2017). A member of the Marketing committee explained:

> There's a study that was done ... that basically shows health practitioners and nutritionists, their rating of the nutritional value of different foods. And then it's compared to what consumers rate as being nutritionally good for you. And almonds rank up in the very top righthand quadrant, #2 on the list. So that information told us that this health message was resonating with the consumers and being reinforced by the nutritionists out there and we really didn't feel a compelling reason to continue to emphasize it .... They're all on board, now it's the next chapter, and what do we say about the product without losing touch with what got us there.

Successful advertising, this interviewee reminded me, is about the cumulative effect of a consistent message over time. Building on existing health messages would have a greater impact than starting from scratch. His explanation of the pivot from disease prevention toward vitality reveals three key dynamics. First, the industry had reached saturation with existing health messages at the same moment when surpluses loomed, requiring a new strategy for driving consumption. Second, investment in nutrition research and messaging created a sense of path-dependency because consistent messages are more cost effective. This resonates with Harvey's theorization of fixity wherein prior investments limit mobility by rooting an industry to a certain space, in this case a semiotic space. Third, through decades of sustained nutrition research, the almond industry had successfully shifted a critical portion of its advertising message over to health professionals and nutritionists who would likely continue working to their benefit at very little expense.

Consumers do not uncritically adopt the health messages offered by nutrition research and industry, yet health has been such a successful advertising platform that the ABC now uses receptivity to health messages, as well as snacking behavior, as the primary criterion for selecting which new countries they will enter. To continue growing consumption in the United States, however, almonds had to do more than sustain health or prevent disease; they needed to surpass the status quo. Under the new wellness and vitality mandate, the committee began funding research on cognitive performance, "skin health" (more accurately, wrinkle prevention), and optimizing gut function. Meanwhile the Marketing committee and its contracted advertising firm had been gradually shifting the advertising message from healthy lifestyles to something more ambitious.

Advertisers increasingly positioned almonds as the source of endless energy required for a non-stop action-packed lifestyle. The advertising team "determined our primary target to be productive to the extreme, driven by their desire to accomplish a seemingly endless number of tasks in a day" (Sterling-Rice Group 2018). In an interview the marketing director told me "for some people that life would feel very frenzied and out of whack, but for this consumer they love it." Presenting a less optimistic take, marketers at the annual industry conference described "one major force shaping snacking habits are the stress levels of younger generations," with an accompanying bar graph showing progressively greater stress ratings between generations X, Y, and Z. They quoted focus group participants describing a "hectic lifestyle" and wishing there were more hours in the day. Almond advertisers want these potential customers to "think of [almonds] as not just the best snack choice but the snack that would give them the energy to keep powering through" (Sterling-Rice Group 2018).

The ABC website identifies ten unique almond snacking occasions as moments of self-regulation amid a white-collar working woman's demanding day: the recovery, the morning prep, the crunch-time rush, the mid-morning battle, the salad plus-up, the chip switch, the afternoon lull, the on-the-goer, the trail mixer, and the late-nighter (Almond Board of California 2018). The accompanying narrative describes almonds as the snack solution for a life of vigorous early morning exercise, constant errands, shuttling children to-and-fro, eating at a desk or while walking, moderating meals, and curbing cravings. While the ABC has chosen not to use the term "superfood" in ads, fearing it might connote a fad, they support the widespread acclaim almonds have received as a nutrition "powerhouse." In 2018, Blue Diamond embraced the superfood attribution by adopting the slogan "Don't deny your cravings. Eat them. All the flavors you crave … in a superfood." At the annual conference, marketers explained it would be most efficient and effective to shift the group of "medium [almond] users" into the category of "heavy users" than to find messages that would attract brand-new almond eaters. While preventative-health framing of almonds emphasized restraint and acquiescence to expertise, the superfood era encourages health-conscious consumers to subtly challenge dietary recommendations and see themselves as potentially unlimited.

Shifts in the advertising strategy accompanying the almond industry's transition from "health" to "vitality" paint a vivid portrait of how the superfood concept reshapes expectations of wellness from disease prevention to hyper productivity. In 2017, advertisers shifted from positioning almonds as an ingredient in a healthy lifestyle to a means for maximizing output. The "Carpe PM" marketing campaign satirized afternoon fatigue as a dire medical condition instantaneously alleviated by the first taste of an almond. While intended to be humorous, the campaign medicalized even the slightest fluctuations in energy, rendered workers responsible for fatigue, and encouraged consumers to see eating almonds as a source of renewed potential. The 2018 "Own Your Everyday" campaign featured the power of almonds to not only alleviate, but enchant the most minute frustrations of a privileged life, such as helping one's husband find the TV remote or changing the office printer's toner cartridge with a swivel of the hips. In each vignette of the series, an "Almond Snacker" introduces a surreal moment of productivity-enhancing enlightenment, infusing trivial decisions with the potential for grandeur. The superfood framing of almonds instructs eaters that if they make the right eating choices, they can not only meet but exceed expectations while making magic of the mundane.

Superfood as Spatial Fix

As almond production swells, the industry must constantly work to shift the way consumers see almonds, from seasonal specialty to superfood. To accomplish this transition, the industry must also work to change the way consumers see themselves, from sophisticated to superhuman. At each narrowly averted crisis of overproduction, a new type of imagined subject emerges. In the early twentieth century, it was a woman seeking to become more modern by letting go of traditional seasonal eating patterns. Throughout the mid-century, almond marketers envisioned a government official or homemaker eager to apply scientific rationale to strengthen the national body. In the 1980s, almond ads evoked a sense of rural nostalgia and civic duty to support American farmers through regular purchasing habits. During the turn of the twenty-first century, almond marketers depicted consumers eager to avoid diet-related diseases through informed food choices. Now, as this market for preventative health offers little room for expansion, they envision women striving to maximize productivity in each minute moment with boundless energy. At each stage, the subjectivity of the eater is reimagined to suit the needs of a spatial fix to chronic agricultural surplus.

Understanding the spatial fix as material *and* semiotic illuminates the importance of meaning-making practices to political economic patterns. Harvey theorized the spatial fix as a temporary solution that functions much like the fleeting fix of addiction. While he treats space as a material configuration, a parallel pattern is evident in the shifting configuration of meanings. Just as markets can be saturated, meanings can be saturated. They are inseparable. Harvey highlights the tension between capital's need for mobility and the fixedness of necessary material infrastructures in a specific location. Likewise, the almond case reveals this tension occurring through meanings. Expanding markets requires new meanings and yet to be effective, advertisers cannot stray far from existing investments in historically cultivated meanings and the semiotic infrastructure of scientifically legitimated nutrition claims.

It is well known that the state enables spatial fixes to agrarian capitalism. Export subsidies, public university research to intensify production, and infrastructures of commodity circulation all facilitate a material reordering of agriculture that can temporarily alleviate overproduction. Far less recognized is the state's role in enabling the accompanying semiotic shifts.

As the almond case demonstrates, state-mandated payments to the ABC have been essential to the industry's ability to execute sophisticated advertising campaigns, fund nutrition research, and advocate for recognized health labels. While early cooperation prior to the federal marketing order propelled the industry's profitability, mandated payments enabled an explosion of marketing activity. US-grown produce rising to superfood status through state- supported overproduction thus carries a distinct trajectory from exotic superfood imports such as quinoa or moringa.

Advertisers often describe themselves as simply identifying existing needs and positioning their product as fulfilling these needs. The historical shifts in almond advertising undoubtedly reflect far-reaching and well-documented social phenomena: the promotion of modernity, the expanded authority of science in domestic activities, growing concern over heart disease and obesity, and the physical and psychological strain of mounting expectations for working women. Yet advertising is not just any mirror to societal change. It is a funhouse mirror, warped along multiple axes to magnify desire.

In the case of almonds, superfood status extends beyond touting the health-promoting chemical composition of a food. It fosters a consumer culture in which food is a coping mechanism for life in overdrive. This resonates with analyses of the neoliberal entrepreneurial self as governed by ambition, calculation, autonomy, and an unrelenting expectation of self-improvement (Brown 2003; Rose 1992; Scharff 2016). Superfood eaters are encouraged to see food as fuel and themselves as engines of productivity with perpetually unmet potential. While preventative health messaging advocated self-management, it lacked the entrepreneurial emphasis on maximizing output. Even the language of cravings and constant snacking amplifies a vision of the self as simultaneously self-regulating and insatiable.

The recent turn toward a superfood framing does not rewrite the many existing meanings ascribed to almonds by consumers: it is merely the semiotic frontier. People may seek out almond products as a substitute for animal protein motivated by environmental or health concerns, or because they are a staple of family recipes, or for other complex motivations an in-depth consumer study might reveal. Marketers do not expect all almond eaters to adopt the hyper-productive subjectivities of superfood eaters, but they do see this vitality message as the growth edge of the industry. Superfood status for the almond industry is a spatial fix, an ever-incomplete process of prolonging agrarian capitalism despite repeated crises of overproduction. As this case demonstrates, the food meanings forged at such frontiers of accumulation carry lasting cultural implications and yet are always destined to be refashioned.

Analyzing a single commodity carries obvious limits, and this work would be greatly enhanced by similar analyses of domestic foods gaining superfood acclaim. Tracing a single commodity historically, however, reveals how intimately agrarian political economy and food culture are knitted together through time. Chronic overproduction, coupled with state-facilitated cooperation and marketing, has pursued spatial fixes, which reshape flows of food materials and meanings alike. As the array of products marketed as superfoods expands, it is worth asking for whom superfoods are ultimately so "super."

Acknowledgements

This chapter is reproduced by permission from Springer Nature: Reisman, E. "Superfood as spatial fix: the ascent of the almond." *Agric Hum Values* 37, 337–351 (2020). https://doi.org/10.1007/s10460-019-09993-4.

Notes

1   Argan oil use for culinary, cosmetic, and medical use is rising rapidly (Grand View Research 2016), largely justified by phytochemical properties analogous to other superfoods, including antioxidants and omega-3 fatty acids. This case demonstrates how superfood status can carry over to multiple pathways of bodily absorption, including both ingestion and topical application, and straddle the line between food and medicine (Loyer 2016b).
2   Estimated $11.14 million (1995 crop of 557.1 million lbs at 0.2/lb), of which at least 60 percent was likely intended for advertising.

3

"The New Pomegranate": Rooibos Magic, Traditional Knowledge, and the Politics and Possibilities of Superfoods

Sarah Ives

Science Has Proven It—Rooibos Tea Is Magic.

(Ebrahim 2016)

Headline after headline extols the "Rooibos Miracle." Exported to more than thirty countries, South African rooibos tea is celebrated for its "earthy" flavor and medicinal qualities. The list of the tea's wonders appears endless: it will help you lose weight, gain weight, and control diabetes; it will promote longevity, make skin more youthful, cure acne, prevent cancer and Parkinson's disease, protect the liver, improve fertility, soothe colicky babies, promote sleep, and provide emotional comfort. Marketing materials describe it as a leading example of a global "superfood." In 2016, *Time Magazine* labeled rooibos one of "The 50 Healthiest Foods of All Time" (Sifferlin 2016). These exhortations have led to a swell of interest in the plant and its bioactive compounds. Rooibos has become a US$22.2 million industry; it constitutes 10 percent of the global herbal tea market and more than 30 percent of South Africa's tea market (Wynberg 2017). According to a 2018 survey of 1,000 South Africans, half drink rooibos every day. Overall, 84 percent said they drink the tea for its health benefits, and 31 percent said drinking it brings back memories of family and friends (South African Food Review 2018).

Food scholar Michael Carolan (2011) writes that "food has always come with a story, which in part explains its power to produce and reproduce culture and identity" (29). The industrialization of food production has led to a sharp reduction of the global population employed in agriculture. As our physical, embodied relationship to food has shifted, Carolan explains, "so too have these stories. Many people, after all, still go to the grocery store looking for a good story" (32; see also Guthman this volume). Like other products, the rooibos "story" varies depending on who is telling it—or who is listening. Rooibos is cultivated almost exclusively where it also grows wild: South Africa's Western and Northern Cape provinces. Some marketing narratives celebrate the plant's ecological indigeneity and its "natural" home among photogenic mountains. Other narratives describe tea growers, their images curated to make them palatable to international consumers searching for an "authentic Africa." Within South Africa, the rooibos story often involves hospitality and national identity; when guests enter a South African home, hosts typically offer rooibos alongside "English" tea. In the growing region, farmers exalt rooibos as an integral part of their heritage and sense of belonging. Many argue that cultivating and drinking rooibos involve more than earning a livelihood; rather, rooibos informs "who we are."

Despite the legion of narratives, the rooibos industry has poured money into finding still more ways to market the tea. In a never-ending search for new consumers, the South African Rooibos Council has contributed R30 million (over US$2 million) in the last decade to research on the plant's health benefits. This funding has coincided with a marketing push that celebrates rooibos *not* as an indigenous plant or as South Africa's national beverage, but *solely* for its superfood health claims. These claims focus on the plant's bioactive compounds operating at the epigenetic level in the consumer's body (see Spackman, this volume).

What are the consequences of re-signifying rooibos—a plant already loaded with semiotic meaning—as a superfood? And what does a shift to thinking about food-as-compound mean for politics in the growing region? Superfood marketing evokes ideas of bodily health and emotional "self-care." Like marketers, residents of the growing area "ascribe a metaphysical quality to rooibos" (Ives 2017, 22). Unlike marketers' emphasis on the body, however, residents include the "holy act" of cultivation in the tea's magic. Rooibos is nature and God's gift to the region. As one grower described, "My heart is rooibos ... My blood is in the soil" (Ives 2014, 707).

Miraculous and inalienable: rooibos infuses the essence of producers who see their blood as part of the soil and consumers who are told that the tea will permeate their bodies at the cellular level. In this sense, superfoods such as rooibos do not fit squarely with the concept of commodity. Marx (1990 [1887]) describes commodities as social phenomena bequeathed with thing-like status and sold on the market. While rooibos may be sold on the market, its associations with magic cause it to transcend the status of being merely "thing-like." The stakes of rooibos's magic, however, are different for well-heeled consumers searching for the next food trend than they are for laborers working in rooibos fields. Tracing global flows involves "more than connecting dots on the map," but also tracing the flow of affect (Fischer and Benson 2006, 5). Indeed, marketers divorce the magic of superfoods from conventional understandings of place. The place that counts in superfood marketing is the body of the consumer.

Marketers depict rooibos's antioxidants as turning back the ravages of aging and fighting many ailments. Yet in a shift away from community-supported agriculture, terroir, or fair-trade discourses, many products marketed as superfoods, such as blueberries, salmon, and kale, do not draw on the location of cultivation to generate their power. Anthropologists Edward Fischer and Peter Benson (2006) describe the "double-commodity fetish" of food. People want to be ignorant about some aspects of food production (a kind of deliberate fetishism), but they are also captivated by the lore of food origins (Cook and Crang 1996; Guthman 2009). While some superfood marketing conjures images of the food as "super" in its health claims *and* in its effects on producers and/or local environments, if food origins emerge at all in rooibos superfood marketing, they are typically relegated to the margins of the story. In stark contrast, place is fundamental to how growers see rooibos. For them, rooibos is a means to assert their heritage in the region.

While political economic investigations of food often explore how capitalism veils exploitation, I focus less on the movement of the plant along a commodity chain than on the translation of rooibos from one "form" to another. By translation, I do not mean the harvesting and processing of the plant as it shifts from bush to tea. Rather, I am interested in how rooibos moves in and out of commodity form, what happens during the process of translation, and whose voices are included (or marginalized) (see Appadurai 1986; Kopytoff 1986). As rooibos circulates, the plant changes from "more than a commodity" to a commodity to "more than a commodity" once again. In the growing region, rooibos is an indigenous plant central to contested claims to belonging. As the tea is packaged and transported, it transforms into an alienated object, disconnected from an intimate relationship with growers and its indigenous ecosystem. When rooibos reaches cups around the world, superfood marketing claims mutate it once again, this time into a meaningful, magical substance that fuses with the consumer's body. Anna Tsing (2015) describes this translation as "the hours that count … the creation of capitalist value from noncapitalist value regimes" (128). In the "hours that count"—or the moments when rooibos takes its commodity form—growers, corporations, the South African government, and those who assert themselves as the original inhabitants of the region struggle over rightful ownership of rooibos's traditional knowledge (TK) and the financial benefits that accrue from it.

To explore rooibos magic and the politics of superfoods, I draw on more than ten years of engagement with the region, including ethnographic research with producers, marketers, scientists, and other industry players. I combine ethnographic work with analysis of rooibos marketing materials and government documents relating to rooibos access and benefit-sharing (ABS). While discussions of commodities often use production as the "start" of the commodity's life, I begin in the "place" where rooibos superfood marketing begins: the body of the consumer. I consider how superfood health claims emphasize ideas of "knowing" the body over "knowing" the location of cultivation, and I address how conceptualizing food as "bioactive compounds" can influence regional politics and the relationship between food, people, and place. In the second section, I shift my attention to the politics of this "knowing" in the growing region in connection to struggles over who can claim TK. Growers who identify as coloured[1] do not fit easily into palatable consumer narratives of indigenous farming communities or into the South African San and Khoi-San Councils, organizations which assert an ethnic indigeneity in relation to rooibos even while their members do not reside in the growing region.

I conclude by bringing the two sides of the rooibos narrative together. In the translation from plant to superfood, marketing shifts attention from the intimate act of living with and growing rooibos to a notion of TK that is disarticulated from the intimate, embodied act of growing the tea in its indigenous ecosystem. By exploring the implications of superfood marketing narratives as they circulate back to sites of cultivation, I show how this translation appears to create space for new claims to rooibos ownership, a space with repercussions for politics *and* financial benefits. These politics—and different understandings of rooibos's magic—hinge on local struggles over rooibos's heritage, authenticity, and contested definitions of TK.

Superfoods, Magic, and the Body

A Google search of the terms "rooibos" and "cure all" returns over 2 million results, with links to sites telling readers to "Drink it up. The health benefits of rooibos tea are endless" (Nkosi 2018). An article aimed at "existing and aspirant" South African businesspeople highlights rooibos's supposed benefits in a litany of alliteration: "silky skin," "healthy hair," "body-booster," "stomach-soother," "bold breathing," and "blood-flow benefits" (ibid.). With each of these claims comes a discussion of the tea's active, natural chemical properties. Its antioxidants (aspalathin and nothofagin) purportedly boost the immune system, fight cancer, and control or prevent diabetes. The article echoes an ever-growing corpus: rooibos is anti-inflammatory, antiviral, antiaging, antibacterial, and antispasmodic.

Imbuing goods with mystical properties is not new or unique. Social theorists often talk about consumption in relation to what it "evokes"—whether it's Bourdieu's notion of class distinction or Proust's ideas of remembrance (Groeniger et al. 2017; Lizie 2013). Consider, for example, the South Africans who drink rooibos to reminisce about family and friends. Interdisciplinary scholars Grasseni et al. (2014) specifically explore the different valuations that accompany food stories. They ask what makes food "good," "better," or "bad." According to the authors, answers vary and depend on consumer ideas about flavor, affordability, accessibility, authenticity, social justice, environmental sustainability, and political empowerment.

But how do these valuations apply to food deemed better than "good"? What about foods that are "super"? While no official definition for superfoods exists, the term implies that the food has a miraculous quality that could relate to health, the environment, and/or various political and economic benefits. The marketing of rooibos as a superfood, however, focuses on the American Heart Association (2018) understanding of the term: foods that are rich in antioxidants and associated with antiaging health claims (Lunn 2006). In the case of rooibos, the miraculous quality stems from how the food acts in (or on) the consumer's body. Envisioning rooibos as a superfood can evoke images of the plant's bioactive components swimming through the body in a superhero cape, battling inflammation, viruses, aging, and even negative emotions.

Labeling a product "super" is good for business. For example, blueberry sales reportedly doubled between 2005 and 2007 after superfood claims (Curll et al. 2016). Shifting rooibos's market narrative in this direction was a conscious decision by industry groups: "Rooibos research has reached a critical point where significant investment is required to take it to the next phase, which is likely to pave the way for other important findings and the possible development of nutraceutical products in combatting disease," Ernest du Toit, spokesperson of the Rooibos Council, stated in a press release (South African Rooibos Council 2019). In other words, the shift toward superfood health claims followed classic capitalist notions of the constant search for—and creation of—new markets. To take rooibos "to the next phase," marketers sought to link it to consumer trends as part of a strategy that includes moving beyond tea through rooibos-infused alcohol, rooibos powders as sports recovery drinks, and an expansion of rooibos skincare lines. Ironically, in using new food technologies to create rooibos extracts, the amount of rooibos in a product *decreases* just as the symbolic attention to the plant *increases* (see Brondizio 2008 for a similar discussion relating to açaí). This marketing is aimed not only at international customers, but also at consumers within South Africa. If half of South Africans already drink rooibos every day, how can marketers get them to consume *even more*?[2]

With its role in traditional Chinese medicine, tea has a long medicinal history, making its marketing as a beverage/medicine seamless. Today marketers often portray tea as a form of self-care. Narratives describe curling up with a cup of tea. There are even flavors for sale dubbed "Snuggle up Tea." Tea bags include tags with inspirational messages such as "Recognize that you are the truth"; "I am beautiful, I am bountiful, I am blissful"; or simply, "Be yourself."[3] Interdisciplinary scholars Curll et al. (2016) argue that "the contemporary high-income consumer is looking for a combination of self-care and social meaning in the food they buy" (92; see also MacGregor et al. 2018). They describe anthropologist Jane Fajans's observation that superfoods

> could become a kind of balm for millennial anxieties ... a miracle cure for, among other things, obesity, attention-deficit disorder, autism, arthritis, Alzheimer's disease, and erectile dysfunction ... it takes away the toxicity of living in the First World and transports you back to the healthy, natural world of the rainforest.
>
> (Ibid.)

This journey, however, does not always evoke a specific place, even as it claims to "transport" consumers. Richard Wilk (2006) notices a similar pattern in a discussion of Fuze, a vitamin-enriched tea and fruit drink. Rather than telling us where the "exotic" juices come from,

> the writing in the bottle is all about the powers of the ingredients to "increase energy levels" and "relieve stress and tension." Instead of telling us who made the ingredients, the bottle uses their foreign names to send a more general message that they are powerful because they come from far away places. Distance and mystery are part of the magic trapped in the bottle.

(1)

Certain products associated with the superfoods concept—blueberries, salmon, and kale—do not focus on the mystery of distance or the lore of origins. Instead, they incorporate the most intimate of spaces: the body. Framing superfoods as both exotic and embodied, external and internal, marketers emphasize a different kind of "lore" (or "knowledge"), the lore of bodies under constant threat from free radicals, aging, and oxidative stress. Part of the lore includes the ability to fight these stresses through consumption choices. Discussing ultrasound imaging and the mapping of the human genome, geographers Bruce Braun and Noel Castree describe how "the body is increasingly a 'material-semiotic' object *known* in such ways that it can be changed" (2005, 14, emphasis added; see also Haraway 1997).

What does this shift in scale imply for our understanding of food politics? Scholars have used food to explore articulations among production; consumption; and the social, economic, environmental, and political forces shaping the world (Freidberg 2004; Mintz 1986; West 2012). Tea, in particular, has figured in struggles over colonial and postcolonial representation (Besky 2014; Chatterjee 2001). Jean Baudrillard (1994) argues that marketing replaces objects with their representations. In other words, Baudrillard challenges the materiality of commodity fetishism by shifting attention from the consumption of objects to the consumption of their "meanings." While superfoods' "meanings" are key to their magic, their materiality remains central. However, it is the compounds (the antioxidants)—and not the complete object—that matter.

The focus on compounds alters the relation between product and place and the articulations among production, consumption, and social and political forces. Sociologist Jane Collins (2014) argues that we need to "crack open" commodities

> to recover some of what neoclassical economics makes us forget: living, breathing, gendered, and raced bodies working under social relations that exploit them; bodies living in households with persons who depend on them and on whom they depend; and bodies who enter into the work of making a living with liveliness, creativity, and skill.
>
> (27)

Thoroughly examining superfoods requires "cracking" open the social relations of production, as well as the bodies of consumers and the components of the products themselves. The messages behind superfoods such as rooibos center on how consuming them can alter the body's ecology through a mystical alchemy.

While some of rooibos's benefits remain unproven, scientific studies show that placebo effects can influence health outcomes—magical thinking that comes to life (Kaptchuk and Miller 2015).

The magical thinking draws on a politics of knowledge. Analyzing milk, Atkins (2010) describes technologies, such as chemical analyses, as ways of "knowing" food, a kind of knowing increasingly prominent in discussions of rooibos: "Science Has Proven It—Rooibos Tea Is Magic," one headline reads (Ebrahim 2016). Consumers "know" food because they "know" its bioactive components and the way that its antioxidants act in the human body, not because they know how or where it grows. But this knowing can be vague, unverified, and even skeptical (Loyer 2016c; Scrinis 2013). In this sense, the knowledge politics differ from discussions about how certain epistemic systems claim authority and police professionalism, or even the inequality between "local" and "scientific" knowledge (Wayland 2003). Instead, the "knowledge" that marketers attempt to cultivate is based on individual lifestyle choices. Notably, some marketers refer to genetically modified (GM) foods as superfoods by labeling them "healthier" for consumers than their non-GM counterparts (Le Page 2018).

Yet the magic of rooibos is not relegated to consumption; it also informs relations between the plant and growers in its indigenous ecosystem. In the following section, I consider how the politics of knowledge fostered by superfood marketing circle back to the growing region. In her discussion of matsutake mushrooms, Anna Tsing (2015) describes the "translation" from plant to commodity as its own kind of magic. In rooibos's "hours that count," the tea's magic transforms from growers' intimate relations with plant and place to marketers' fixation on consumers' bodies. The process of translation from plant to superfood, in which knowledge about rooibos's healing properties supplants the significance of rooibos's geographical origins, appears to open a space for new claims to rooibos ownership, a space with repercussions for the politics and possibilities in the growing region.

Between the Field and the Cup: The Politics of Knowledge in South Africa

With rooibos's growing popularity, industry players have attempted to protect, symbolically and legally, its terroir or its unique connection to place. Food scholars argue that as dishes become hybridized and indigenized in new places, producers who consider the food to be "theirs" react with anxiety and endeavor to claim legal ownership through trademarks or Geographic Indications (GIs) (Parasecoli 2017; Paxson 2010). According to the World Intellectual Property Organization (WIPO), GIs are a "sign used on products that have a specific geographical origin and possess qualities or a reputation that are due to that origin." In other words, the WIPO asserts that the product's qualities derive from the "geographical place of production," an assertion that creates an indissociable link between product and place. While recognizing that these claims have an economic basis, historian Ari Ariel (2012) argues that "more than this, however, it is part of a larger effort at preserving the imagined uniqueness of ethnic and national groups in the face of the perceived threat of others, and an attempt to concretize and legalize the amorphous concept of authenticity" (35). The rooibos industry attempted to "concretize" the plant's ecological "authenticity" in its indigenous landscape through a successful bid for a GI in 2014 (Coombe et al. 2015). Labels such as GIs and Fair Trade are designed to foster consumer beliefs that their purchases make the places where products originate somehow better; the labels seem to bring nonmarket values into markets (Besky 2014).

The language around superfoods complicates the significance of this protection in relation to marketing claims that focus entirely on health. Alongside its successful campaign for a GI, industry players also fought an attempt by Nestlé to patent research results relating to "consumer benefits" from rooibos extracts. Instead of bioprospecting the *plant*, Nestlé argued that it was patenting its *research findings*. In some respects, the fact that the rooibos industry was able to fight Nestlé's patent appears to reinforce South Africa's claims to the plant and the knowledge surrounding it. South African media sources largely portrayed the outcome as a win for the country, as reclaiming the country's heritage from "Corporate Food." However, superfood marketing's emphasis on bioactive ingredients instead of on rooibos in its own right speaks to Nestlé's larger framing of knowledge and consumer benefit: Nestlé spokespeople described rooibos patents as part of the company's research program in bioactive ingredients. Indeed, in 2018 Nestlé announced that it was partnering with the company, Nuritas, to use a "data-driven approach," including artificial intelligence and DNA, to discover bioactive peptide networks within natural food sources (Nuritas 2019). The natural food sources were unnamed: it was not the food source that was key to this new technological understanding of food, but the peptides.

Similarly, in rooibos superfood marketing, where the plant comes from is of only minor significance: what matters are the charisma of the plant's chemistry and the story of what it does for your body. Instead of focusing on authenticity of production, superfood *health* claims are policed by the European Union and the US Food and Drug Administration. If the superfood designation stems from antioxidants' cancer-fighting properties, then the rooibos miracle could be replaced when a new "super" product reaches stores. Ultimately, marketing narratives that favor *compounds* over the entirety of *plants* are stories of commensurability and exchangeability, such that if another product contains a better ratio of the compounds than rooibos does, the unique value of rooibos as a superfood could be lost.

The magic of consuming rooibos is far less interchangeable for growers, who sometimes feed their babies rooibos alongside breast milk, a deeply embodied connection between grower, plant, and place. In one sense, growers are not completely distinct from international consumers. They express belief in rooibos's magical abilities to act on the body by soothing babies and improving health and wellbeing. Yet they describe an intimacy in their daily, embodied relationship with the tea *beyond* the extraction of value for the market. In de-emphasizing the location of cultivation, however, superfood marketing shifts attention from the intimate act of living with and growing rooibos to a more disembodied—or "entirely intangible"—notion of TK.

Conflicts over TK and indigeneity derive in part from the rooibos-growing region's history. For millennia, the area was inhabited by hunter-gatherers (often referred to as "San"). During the first millennium AD, herders (often referred to as "Khoi") introduced pastoralism (Penn 2005). Europeans arrived in the mid-seventeenth century, leading to the dispossession and decimation of the San and Khoi populations through violent conquest and disease. Conquest included murder, enslavement, and rape, as well as theft of livestock and other means of livelihood, thereby forcing the Khoisan[4] into labor or into moving north as the colonial frontier pushed up the continent. The cumulative effect was the virtual genocide of the Khoisan in the region (Adhikari 2010).

This history sheds light on contemporary racial dynamics in South Africa that are often erased by a settler/native, white/black binary, a binary reinforced by apartheid's codified racial and ethnic groupings. Rooibos is endemic, but most people who cultivate the plant today do not claim a Khoisan heritage. While South Africa is classified as 81 percent black, 9 percent coloured, 8 percent white, and 2 percent Asian, the growing region is approximately 80 percent coloured, 15 percent white, and 5 percent black (Statistics South Statistics South Africa 2017). Unlike the racial "purity" associated with the term "black" in South Africa, the term "coloured" refers to people from a heterogeneous combination of heritages, including those from the Khoisan community, people of biracial heritage, and people brought as slaves or laborers from other African countries and from regions such as Southeast Asia (Adhikari 2005; Jensen 2008). Supposedly born out of rape and miscegenation, coloured people are often framed as indigenous to nowhere and envisioned as having a false identity that lacks a precolonial reality.

Yet coloured residents forged their belonging in the region in part through their espoused cultural ownership of indigenous, magical rooibos (Ives 2017). Rooibos was more than a plant or a tea: they believed it was their heritage. Their collective memories were formed through and with the rooibos landscape, even if land ownership remained largely out of reach. Although white residents comprise only 15 percent of the population, they own 93 percent of rooibos land (Sandra Kruger and Associates 2009). The stakes of rooibos knowledge ownership are high for coloured farmers. Rooibos provides hope for livelihoods in a country where they are often deemed neither white enough nor black enough to make claims to land, resources, or an authentic heritage.

A New Geography of Knowledge?

Recently, contestations over rooibos's heritage have expanded beyond growers— *they have extended to people who do not live in the region at all.* The South African San Council and National Khoi-San Council are negotiating a benefit-sharing agreement with the rooibos industry. Drawing from international precedents, South Africa developed a Biodiversity Act in 2004. The act mandates that anyone "bioprospecting" an indigenous biological resource or the associated "traditional knowledge" must apply for a permit. The Department of Environmental Affairs (DEA) states that "Local traditional knowledge (TK) of the value and use of biological resources is unique to a culture or society and is passed from generation to generation through word of mouth and cultural rituals. This TK is usually built by a group of people living in close contact with nature" (2014, 1). The department provides three key characteristics for this knowledge: It "has been created over a long period of time, passed down from generation to generation; is constantly improved as new knowledge is integrated to the existing; and the creation and improvement of knowledge is a group effort" (3).

In 2010, the South African San Council (whose members live outside the rooibos region) sent a letter to the director general of Environmental Affairs asserting that the San are the primary knowledge holders of rooibos (among other native species) and that they should therefore receive financial benefits from its sale (Wynberg 2017). In 2013, the National Khoi-San Council joined the San Council's claim "to establish a negotiating body [on] behalf of all San and Khoi Khoi peoples in South Africa" in relation to "their traditional knowledge and associated intellectual property rights" regarding rooibos. The councils followed the precedent set by similar claims involving hoodia, a desert plant that grows to the north of the rooibos region. While the San Council made a successful claim to hoodia, direct monetary benefits were never realized, as hoodia proved less marketable than anticipated after scientific studies seemed to undermine its health benefits (Foster 2017; Wynberg et al. 2009).

Notably, in the cases of both hoodia and rooibos, San Council claims did not include a restoration of land rights lodged with the Commission on Restitution of Land Rights. In other words, the council was not asking to take possession of the land on which the plants grow; instead, they were asserting that they are the original owners of the traditional *knowledge* of the plants. While work in environmental anthropology often addresses how collective memories are read through and with landscapes (Basso 1996; Dove 2011), the council argues only that its members should receive financial benefits from the plant's sale—even if those members do not cultivate rooibos. According to a lawyer involved in the negotiations, "the San declared that they were the original people and therefore the original [TK] holders." In other words, the San Council claimed a forgotten knowledge about rooibos's magical properties, a knowledge that was destroyed when they were separated from the land, *but a knowledge that is traditional nevertheless*. In this sense, rooibos's magic would involve (re)connecting council members to a region where they have been "absent" for hundreds of years.[5] The council is asking to be a stakeholder on the grounds that the San contributed to the use of rooibos because they were the original knowledge holders of its miracle-like properties. The letter written on their behalf stated:

> the San, as "primary knowledge holders" … [should] be formally acknowledged as "stakeholders" within the meaning of the Act, as an indigenous community whose "traditional uses" of the indigenous biological resources have initiated or contributed towards the current bioprospecting.
>
> (Chennells Albertyn 2010; cited in Wynberg 2017, 41)

This magic relies on an idea of rooibos that is more than a commodity, but one that focuses on intangible knowledge and not on an embodied relationship with the land (or even current knowledge about the plant, its cultivation, or its medicinal properties). The government recognized the claim in 2014. In the agreement signed in 2019, the parties established that the councils would receive 1.5 percent of rooibos's "Farm Gate Price" (or the invoiced price paid by processors to farmers for the purchase of harvested, unprocessed, and/or fermented and dried rooibos, exclusive of taxes). Depending on weather and the price of rooibos, among other factors, more than R10 million (or nearly US$700,000) per year could be distributed (Wynberg 2019). The money is to go to a trust, but how that trust will be used and distributed remained unclear at the time of writing.

Through these negotiations, government—and government-recognized, ethnically based councils—appears to determine whose voices are heard and whose voices are marginalized in battles over "knowledge ownership." That said, the agreement stated that there should be "meaningful consultations" with "all rural communities that have traditional knowledge" (Wynberg 2017, 42). In other words, the councils did acknowledge the role of other knowledge holders, such as those in the region's coloured community. The meaning of that consultation and recognition remains unclear; however, in the 2019 agreement these farmers were included under the category, "Rooibos Indigenous Farming Communities." The agreement defines coloured farmers as descendant of the Khoi Khoi, and they are to receive some benefits through the Khoi-San Council.

While benefit-sharing may expand financial rewards beyond white commercial producers, the concept of TK also risks (re)valorizing racial categories perpetuated by apartheid. Definitions of "traditional" in South Africa raise questions in relation to the country's colonial history—the term was weaponized by the apartheid government, which used ideas of "traditional culture" to justify segregation and the relegation of the majority black population to ethnically based *traditional* homelands. Anthropologists, popular culture, and the government mythologized the idea of Khoisan as "traditional," "original people," and a "natural part of the landscape," even as they were dispossessed of their land (Ives 2014; Wilmsen 1989). The idea of indigeneity is also complicated by the region's long histories of migrations and violent dispossessions. Some posit that everyone who is not white is indigenous, while others assert that Khoisan are the only "authentic" indigenous people because they are "the original people" (Meskell 2012). In this understanding, coloured residents seem to count as "indigenous" only if they declare a Khoisan identity.

How does TK function in a region with such a fraught connection to the concept of tradition? Those who claim rooibos TK are reimagining what "traditional belonging" means in a country upended by colonialism and apartheid. While no universally accepted definition of Traditional Ecological Knowledge exists, the concept generally refers to the knowledge acquired by indigenous and local people over hundreds of years through contact with the environment (Berkes 1993). Like the definition used by South Africa's DEA, this widely cited characterization highlights the relationship between living beings with one another and their environment, and it privileges historical continuity in resource-use practices, or "ancient ways of knowing" (2). Historical continuity—or even a close relationship with the environment— complicates the San Council and National Khoi-San Council's claims. Leaders of the councils do not live in the rooibos region and have no living memory of cultivating rooibos. At its founding, the South African San Council represented communities spread across the northern part of the country, including more than 4,000 people who had been resettled from Namibia and Angola. Today, South African law requires the councils to hold regular elections for leaders based on formal written constitutions. Yet this kind of leadership is a modern phenomenon: prior to these regulations, the San did not acknowledge individual leaders. Indeed, the South African Human Rights Commission reported that "reinventing a community from dispersed San descendants was one of the major challenges this community had to face" (Wynberg et al. 2009, 9).

How does their lack of embodied labor in a particular landscape coincide with their TK claims? According to Marx (1990 [1887]), a commodity's exchange value corresponds to the amount of labor time involved in producing it. In other words, commodities embody labor power. In the context of this embodiment, Marx introduces his definition of commodity fetishism: that value inheres in commodities themselves, rather than being added through labor. Fetishism elides the labor power, alienation, and exploitation behind the commodity.

Rooibos as a superfood muddies this concept by emphasizing the role of knowledge over the role of labor. On the one hand, San and Khoi-San Council assertions of ownership without labor could appear to be a form of commodity fetishism. Yet the councils articulate a form of alienation that denies the possibility of labor: complete dispossession. Cecil Le Fleur, chair of the National Khoi-San Council, stated that the government's granting of rooibos TK ownership to the council was important not only for financial benefits but for "the recognition of the Khoi and San people as a people, as a people who had this relationship with the Cederberg mountains" (Vollenhoven 2018).

The dearth of documented evidence about what the Khoisan did and did not know about rooibos complicates how to define and "authenticate" traditional rooibos knowledge prior to European colonization. In research sponsored by the industry-affiliated South African Rooibos Council, Boris Gorelik (2017) attempts to find "verifiable facts" about precolonial rooibos use in order to determine the "truth" about rooibos TK. Perhaps predictably, he was unable to find "sufficient record that would allow us to attribute the origins of traditional knowledge associated with rooibos to any particular community or population group" (48). How does TK account for communities who were dispossessed of their land and resources hundreds of years prior? Wynberg (2017, 42) highlights the tension between "achieving historical and restorative justice for the San and Khoi and recognizing the many others who have provided knowledge towards the success of the rooibos industry." These "many others" include local coloured farmers who have worked with rooibos for generations and feel that the plant and tea are their cultural heritage.

The Stakes of Rooibos Access and Benefit Sharing

"They started the business with the knowledge from us," a coloured farmer asserted, a knowledge he felt remained unacknowledged and a knowledge many felt had been stolen by the largely white tea industry and commercial farmers (Ives 2017, 92). Coloured farmers argued that knowledge about finding seeds, cultivating and processing plants, and even rooibos's medicinal properties came from their community (Keahey 2013). On learning about the councils' claim to rooibos's TK, some coloured growers in the region expressed confusion—and at times anger. Uncertain about what the councils' TK claims would mean for them, many coloured growers found themselves left out of the story because they did not have an "authentic" cultural heritage. "To top it off," the farmer continued, "the Khoisan now declare that they want to benefit! Our people ... are the ones who collect seed. Are we going back to the old South Africa where people are classed by race? I don't know where I belong—black, white, coloured?" (Wynberg 2017, 46).

In April 2018, I attended a meeting in the heart of rooibos country about ABS. For two days, farmers, researchers, industry members, representatives of non-governmental organizations, and others met in the back room of a restaurant housed in an old Masonic lodge. As we talked during formal presentations and informal meals and tea breaks, many coloured farmers expressed that the government negotiations were not acknowledging their voices—or their identities. The goal of the workshop was to provide a platform to share research and development on access and benefit sharing in the Western Cape more generally, but the focus quickly turned to rooibos. Because no one who was party to the ongoing negotiations could talk about the specifics, more questions were raised than answers provided. A lawyer involved attempted to address some concerns when coloured farmers asked how they could get logistical support to be officially recognized as rooibos TK holders. He responded that they needed to contact the leadership of the National Khoi-San Council. "But *we* kept the rooibos tradition alive," someone interjected. "What about us?"

The lawyer assured coloured famers that they would benefit, but the process remains uncertain to this day. At the same time, the meeting prompted reflection among the coloured farming community about their relation to the Khoisan. One person commented, "The grouping of 'coloured people'—they were not born, they were created—white folks grouped all brown-skinned people together and labelled them 'coloureds.' Now it is up to us to decide who or what we are." The lawyer appeared to agree. "You don't have to say you are Khoi," he stated. "You should be able to self-identify however you want." Yet the 2019 agreement and a 2018 documentary, "Rooibos Restitution," suggest otherwise. Rather than embracing the idea of coloured identity and heritage with rooibos, the film suggests that members of the coloured community are (re)envisioning themselves as Khoisan. In one scene, the head of a rooibos cooperative asks a young man: "If someone tells you you're coloured, how do you feel about that?" He responds, "Previously I could accept it, but now that I know where I belong ... " The other youth in the room concurs: "I am a Khoi, and I am proud of that" (Vollenhoven 2018).

Despite assurances that community members could identify how they choose, the idea of TK hinged on the word "tradition," and tradition required a reckoning with the past, a feat that was challenging for many in the region. "A lot of elders don't want to talk about the past, and subtlety and sensitivity is necessary when engaging with the past with the community and within the household," Rhoda Malgas said during the ABS meeting. Indeed, ideas of TK can appear to skip the recent past in search of a more straightforward understanding of South African history, a theme echoed in rooibos marketing that erases colonial violence, dispossession, and persistent inequality. The politics of rooibos TK, then, becomes a matter of policing not only ownership and belonging, but also a matter of policing memory, history, *what* counts as evidence, and *who* counts as authentic—all through an idea of knowledge that is disarticulated from the location of cultivation and the intimate, embodied act of growing the tea in its indigenous ecosystem.

Conclusion

Rooibos is "the new pomegranate juice."

(Grose 2011)

A 2017 survey conducted by the British Nutrition Foundation found that about a third of UK primary students believe cheese comes from plants and pasta comes from meat (British Nutrition Foundation 2017). In response to these trends, movements such as fair trade and community-supported agriculture attempt to reconnect consumers to food production by emphasizing the environment and/or people involved in growing food (Dixon et al. 2014). Rather than (re)connecting consumers to the location of cultivation, however, the rooibos industry's use of superfood marketing stresses the place of the consumer's body. The story that moves to the foreground is that of chemistry and nutritional sciences. In this story, rooibos can be "the new pomegranate"—or the new blueberry, kale, or salmon. The food's value derives from its compounds, not from its unique history or connection to a people or a place.

Despite this suggested replaceability, superfoods do not fit neatly with the concept of commodity. Rooibos consumers *and* producers found a magic more akin to a gift or a totem than to the calculated attributes of a commodity. Marketers described rooibos as redeeming consumer bodies, the antioxidants turning back the ravages of time. Coloured farmers saw rooibos as a means to assert their heritage in the region. The San and Khoi-San Councils sought financial benefits—and perhaps a connection to place. In the process of translation from plant to superfood, knowledge about rooibos's healing properties superseded the significance of rooibos's geographical origins, potentially allowing for new claims to rooibos ownership and its profits. During the "brief hours" of translation, the politics of this knowledge proliferates—whether in the form of scientists and marketers discussing health benefits or in the form of certifying bodies, lawyers, and the government determining ownership of the plant and its magical qualities.

Examining rooibos as a superfood highlights the implications of marketing when the narratives circulate back to locations of cultivation, particularly in the case of indigenous crops viewed as central to understandings of heritage. Marketers' focus on consumer health and knowledge politics also connects to understandings of capital and the (neoliberal) self. In this sense, perhaps rather than being an imperfect fit with the concept of commodity, rooibos emerges as a "super" commodity.

If we understand rooibos as a "super" commodity, another concern emerges: if superfoods represent the latest food trend, what will happen to rooibos when the trend passes? If capitalism rests on the idea of speculation and unending growth, marketers will continue to search for the next thing always over the horizon, something better, something more-than-super. Will demand drop? Or will the rooibos industry adapt and find new markets? What will happen to the knowledge politics? If we follow the example of hoodia, the politics around TK will continue. The San Council gained rights to hoodia, and even though the hoodia market disintegrated, the council persisted in its claims to indigenous resources using the hoodia precedent. For the San Council, the actual plant— rooibos—and its materiality seem tangential to claims to original belonging in South Africa, just as Nestlé could continue its search for bioactive compounds without rooibos. What remains are the people who cultivate rooibos in a region where the tea is consumed alongside breast milk and the senses of belonging and heritage in *this* place with *this* plant are inalienable.

Notes

1   I have maintained the South African spelling of the word to differentiate the term from common understandings in the United States.

2   An interesting parallel emerges with Julie Guthman and Melanie DuPuis's argument in "Embodying Neoliberalism" (2006). The authors describe the bodily contradictions within contemporary capitalism: Companies push consumers to consume more and more while at the same time punishing them if their bodies display signs of "overconsumption" (such as obesity). Rooibos marketing seems to take this contradiction out of the equation. Instead, the marketing pushes people toward the idea that they can never get enough health compounds and must keep searching for new sources to consume ever-more quantities; according to the narrative, it is impossible to overconsume.

3   For more tea bag messages, see Kathy Edwards-Tubbs's Pinterest account, "Messages from My Tea Bags," and other similar social media accounts and blogs.

4   I use the term "Khoisan" to refer to a general idea of the pre-colonial people who lived in the rooibos-growing area, as this was the term most often employed *in* the region. However, distinctions between San, Khoi, and Khoisan exist in relation to how people self-identify *outside* of the region, including the South African San Council and National Khoi-San Council, organizations that claim rooibos knowledge ownership. Because these groups are working together to make their claim, I will not tackle the distinctions here.

5   This discussion has been made more complex by a 2018 documentary, "Rooibos Restitution," which seems to depict local growers as part of the San Council, even though few had heard of the council during the initial negotiations or during the 2018 ABS meeting in Clanwilliam (Vollenhoven 2018).

4

Extractionist Logics: The Missing Link Between Functional Foods and Superfoods

Christy Spackman

"Ready. Easy. Fizzy. Zesty. Pure. Wet. Brisk. Zippy. Tasty."

Filled with colorful bottles, the display case under this line of words at the Union Square Whole Foods in New York City in late 2008 offered to not only assuage thirst, it offered much more. The messages on, and ostensibly the products in, the wide array of bottles promised weight loss, increased brain function, and, most tellingly, the possibility of a dose of antioxidants to take the daily struggle for longevity down to the body's most molecular levels demonstrated through graphs of Oxygen Radical Absorbance Capacity (ORAC). These functional beverages, like their functional food counterparts, promised access to otherwise difficult to access health-promoting molecules via the technological wizardry of industrial food. They offered, in short, hope in a bottle.

Ten years later, a line of messages about the wholeness of the company—from the Whole Kids to the Whole Cities and Whole Planet initiatives—crown the same display case. The messaging shift indexes a change found in the still-present array of colorful bottles promising a better future through consumption. Labels no longer sport graphs of ORAC activity. Rather than discussing how a particular beverage may prevent specific forms of cellular damage caused by invisible molecules, the beverage labels now highlight how their *wholeness* can make a healthier you. Their core ingredients, most of the bottles indicate, are not isolated extractions, but rather superfoods; whole foods commonly used by "traditional cultures" that science has identified as containing high levels of good-for-the-body molecules (Loyer 2016a). The messaging implies that you could easily make these beverages yourself—should you have the inclination and access to the right distribution chains.

This chapter examines how, in the span of a few years, the predominant food-as-medicine discourse shifted from one primarily characterized by nutritional reductionism (Scrinis 2008) to one primarily characterized by wholeness. I investigate the regulatory and technological infrastructures that have facilitated contemporary mobilization of nutritional reductionism in food manufacturing and marketing, infrastructures that pushed industrial logics of molecularization and rebuilding to their most fantastical forms (foods such as pasta fortified with omega-3 fatty acids normally found in fish, for example), and then examine how these infrastructures have entered into the superfood landscape. I focus primarily on the entwining of regulatory and techno-scientific infrastructures in creating what I term "extractionist logics." Extractionist logics refer to the way that nutritional reductionism activates the molecular imagination in researchers, policymakers, food producers, marketers, and eaters in a way that enacts a doubled extraction: first the extraction of molecules from source ingredients/foods; and second, the transformation of eaters into micro-extractors of knowledge and value (energetic, health, social, cultural) from the food choices available to them.

To do this, I first situate functional foods within the larger history of food as medicine. I then examine how techniques in chemistry and biology, developed primarily during the second half of the twentieth century, enabled the rise of an epistemic culture of extraction that contributed to the growth of the functional food market in the United States. I specifically examine the rise and subsequent decline of the ORAC assay as a mode of understanding and communicating molecular materiality across a range of scales. I focus on the ORAC assay for two reasons: it was the first method officially adopted by the Association of Official Agricultural Chemists to measure total antioxidant capacity, and it was the form of measurement commonly mobilized on in-market communication and popular literature during the 2008–12 period. Using Cori Hayden's suggestion that "knowledge and bioartifacts contain, reproduce, or represent people's interests" (Hayden 2003, 19), I explore how identifying and measuring antioxidant activity contained, reproduced, or represented people's interests, a process that allowed extractionist logics to circulate not only beyond the laboratory, but also beyond the functional food landscape they codeveloped with.

Reading through their claims of potential impact on cellular and molecular mechanisms, functional foods exist somewhere between food and medicine. This liminality not only creates spaces of confusion for consumers, it also supports the popularity of the superfood category by facilitating a search for health through foods understood as potentially having therapeutic benefits. How, though, do these foods come to be understood as potentially therapeutic? Writing about pharmaceuticals, Sismondo and Greene note that "bare molecules do not become pharmaceuticals without ties to health concerns, scientific knowledge, appropriate regulation, effective marketing, and receptive prescribers and publics" (Sismondo and Greene 2015, 2). One could make a similar statement with regards to the bioactive molecules found in food: they do not become functionally important micronutrients, nor epigenetically dangerous signals (see Landecker 2011), without ties to health concerns, scientific knowledge, technical practice, regulation, marketing, and receptive publics. By examining how ties between various actors support the emergence and endurance of extractionist logics, we gain an understanding of how science and technology facilitate a certain form of legibility for food— of its core molecular ingredients—that intertwines with market economies in ways that transcend the fashion cycle (Davis 1992). These extractionist logics facilitate what Reisman (this volume), building on Guthman's work (2011), refers to as a "material-semiotic fix," a compilation of meaning that contributes to the continued expansion of certain food markets. As examining extractionist logics in-the-making demonstrates, what appear as food "trends" are rather reflections of social concerns about bodies and health that are deeply rooted in complex relationships between a range of economic, regulatory, and scientific actors.

Methodological Note

This research is based on a dual process of observing physical and epistemic objects. The physical objects I observed were functional beverages, primarily collected by myself and augmented by donations from colleagues from 2008 to 2014, with the bulk of collecting occurring between 2008 and 2012. Now housed at the Southern Food and Beverage Museum, the collection contains more than forty examples of beverages categorized as functional by on-package messaging or advertising. The epistemic objects I observed were much less concrete, in line with Hans-Jorg Rheinberger's definition of epistemic objects as material objects that exceed or transcend efforts to know them, and in the process are continually kept alive as objects of scientific research (Rheinberger 1997, 2005, 406–7). Following Rheinberger, I observed food as it traveled through scientific laboratories and out into the world in the form of publications, regulatory statements, marketing labels, and policies, with a focus on the work produced by the laboratory of Ronald L. Prior at both the United State Department of Agriculture's (USDA) Agricultural Research Service and at the USDA Human Nutrition Research Center on Aging at Tufts University.

Bridging Food and Medicine

From a bird's eye view, the idea that food can act in medicinal ways—that eating certain foods can bring health, wellness, and longevity—underlies both functional foods and superfoods. Thinking of food as medicine is not new. For much of history, food has been one of the core sources of medicine: from the Galenic understanding of foods as balancing humors (Albala 2002; Shapin 2011) to the intimate entwinement of medicinal foods with the Chinese meal structure (Farquhar 2002). In many cases, sensorial perception (touch, taste, smell, sight, texture) played a core role in evaluating the medicinal properties of foods. This relationship between perceptual experience and eating undergirded medical practice in the Western world until the Cartesian Revolution in scientific thinking began to upend the relationship between individual bodies and expertise.

As chemical, mechanical, and biological modes of knowing the world became increasingly accepted over the eighteenth and nineteenth centuries, the authority of individual knowledge about the medicinal uses of food decreased. Physicians in the United States have worked since colonial times to gain control over access to patients and how patients are treated, often by seeking to marginalize treatments and therapies that fall outside of the technological and mechanistic worldview of modern Western medicine (Andrews 1996; Starr 1982). In the early twentieth century, the discovery, purification, and administration of vitamins resulted in theatrical-like demonstrations of the efficacy of nutritional knowledge (Apple 1996). Noticeable improvements in the population's health followed. Mainstream thought, embodied in regulatory policy, came to embrace an understanding of food as a deliverer of molecular entities—macronutrients and micronutrients—that could affect health.

How individuals and institutions in the United States think about health has shifted during the twentieth century. Increasingly, scholars point out, parts of life once considered outside the purview of medicine have been medicalized and, more recently, biomedicalized (Clark et al. 2010). Medicalization is the view that everyday problems and behaviors are things that can be treated by medical intervention; many scholars see this as a central, characterizing aspect of life in the twentieth century. Feeling sad? Take a pill! Biomedicalization, in turn, refers to how technological and scientific knowledge-production infrastructures focused on biological processes (genetics, cell signaling, etc.) have remade medicalization (Clark et al. 2010). Both processes operate by understanding and promoting understandings of bodies as always out of order (Dumit 2012; Nichter and Thompson 2006), something that regularly invites seeking after an idealized, perfect self via consumer activity (e.g., Sikka 2019).

Public and private institutions have not only mobilized market economies to address the body's ills during the twentieth century. They have also mobilized market economies to promote environmental conservation and economic development. Hayden suggests since the 1980s this "paradigm of sustainable development" has led to "nature, as biodiversity ... being framed as a storehouse of valuable genetic resources" (Hayden 2003, 49). Shared between the pharmaceutical industry, biodiversity scientists, and NGOs, efforts to use the market to protect nature manifested as increased attention to molecules found in plants and microbes as potential sources of new medicinal cures (Hayden 2003, 57). Seeing nature as a storehouse of untapped molecules resulted in what many have called bioprospecting, a new manifestation of an ages-old process of extracting plants from one location on the globe and transporting them to other locales for exploitation. Reading nature this way intimately links the natural and technological: one can't understand nature as molecular without analytical instruments that identify molecules.

Like the pharmaceutical sciences, nutritional science sees nature as a storehouse of valuable molecular resources. It is hard from a present-day vantage to fathom a life before food was molecular, before it came with labels telling eaters how much energy each gram could generate, or what percentage of one's recommended daily allowance of vitamins and minerals such a food contained. A reduction to food as composed of molecules that carry different biological impacts undergirds current scientific and social understandings of food; Gyorgy Scrinis terms this approach "nutritionism" (2008). Despite calls by a subset of nutritionists to expand their view (Hoffman 2003), Scrinis argues that nutrition as a field remains focused on the relationship between molecular components found in foods and the corresponding cellular functions of the eating body. Emily Yates-Doerr points out, in her examination of nutritional education in the Guatemalan highlands, that nutritionism creates systematic knowledge about the world; this knowledge can be mobilized to create and enact policy, inform education, and ultimately shape population health (Mudry 2009; Yates-Doerr 2015). Functional foods came into being, especially in the United States, in this cultural milieu where bodies were increasingly understood as at-risk, where health policy and marketing efforts tasked individuals with using market systems to manage their own wellness, and where naturally occurring or chemically manufactured molecules carried the potential to rescue both individual body and world environment.

Regulatory Fences

National regulatory bodies have played a key part in the making of functional foods. As a category, functional foods came into being as part of a Japanese state-sponsored project exploring how food, when twinned with medical science, could be used to "beat life-style related diseases" (Arai 2002, S139; Spackman 2014). Aimed at producing "foods for specified health use," the project sought to address problems such as increases in allergic reactions to foods as well as diseases brought on by ever-increasing lifespans (Swinbanks and O'Brien 1993). The project carried the added bonus of attracting international attention from researchers and food producers.

Loosely defined as "foods that provide a health benefit beyond basic nutrition" (Joy 2007), the functional food category could best be described as one that goes beyond conventional foods. Thus, although as the ADA notes in their 2009 position statement on functional foods that the simplest functional foods are fruits and vegetables (American Dietetic Association 2009), the moniker generally refers to foods "enhanced" or fortified with compounds understood to be biologically active. It is this understanding of parts of food as biologically active—able to reduce inflammation, or improve brain power, for example—that brings functional foods right up to the regulatory line dividing food from medicine and, as such, enters them into entirely new regulatory landscapes.

The unevenness of the regulatory landscape around food marketing in the United States facilitated the growth of functional foods. The functional food category as currently constituted emerged during the deregulatory Reagan era, with the allowance of "health claims without premarket approval" by the Food and Drug Administration (FDA) in 1987 (Heller 2005, 171). Not surprisingly, the number of claims on food labels exploded, with the cover story of *Business Weekly* demanding on October 9, 1989, "Can Corn Flakes Cure Cancer? Of Course Not. But Health Claims for Foods Are Becoming Ridiculous." By 1990, the US Congress responded to calls for reform from consumer advocates, industry players, and regulators by passing the Nutrition Labeling and Education Act (NLEA). NLEA permits health claims that "describe a relationship between a food substance and a disease" and carry the backing of "significant scientific agreement among qualified experts" regarding the validity of the claim (American Dietetic Association 2009). NLEA-approved claims require significant research time and money; currently only twelve types of claims are approved (Center for Food Safety and Applied Nutrition, Office of Nutritional Products, Labeling, and Dietary Supplements 2013). Consider, for example, the claim found on a Bolthouse Farms Heart Healthy Pear Merlot Apple Juice Blend: "Barlive barley betafiber is a natural source of beta-glucan soluble fiber that helps support heart health with 3 g per day, when consumed as part of a low fat, low cholesterol diet. This bottle of juice contains 1.4 g of beta-glucan soluble fiber (0.75 g per 8 oz serving)." This claim is NLEA-approved under 21 CFR 101.81, "Soluble Fiber from Certain Foods and Risk of Coronary Heart Disease." Implementation of NLEA slowed the frenzied business of making health claims on food to an ordered trickle between 1990 and 1994.

Many, especially those in the supplement business, found the NLEA overly constraining, a regulatory dead end that got in the way of consumer choice. In 1994, Congress officially responded to those concerns by passing the Dietary Supplement Health and Education Act (DSHEA) (Apple 1996, 174–7). Supported by both Republicans and Democrats, DSHEA re-opened the door for functional foods by allowing structure/function claims. These claims, unlike those permitted by the NLEA, "describe how a food component or ingredient affects the structure and/or function of the body (e.g., calcium builds strong bones) without linking it to a specific disease" (American Dietetic Association 2009). As long as a food fell into the category of dietary supplement, the claim did *not* need the backing of significant scientific agreement. Supplement users around the country rejoiced.

Further modifications occurred in 1997 under the Food and Drug Administration Modernization Act of 1997, allowing "manufacturers to use health claims if such claims are based on current, published, authoritative statements" from the National Institute of Health, Centers for Disease Control and Prevention, or National Academy of Sciences (American Dietetic Association 2009). Five years later, in 2003, the FDA further loosened regulations by allowing qualified health claims: claims that do not yet meet the standard of significant scientific agreement, but do have some scientific support. Examples of qualified claims include claims linking green tea consumption to decreased risk of cancer and omega-3 fatty acids with a reduced risk of coronary heart disease.

Currently, functional foods, depending on the health claims made and ingredients used in their manufacture, are "regulated as 'foods,' 'dietary supplements,' 'drugs,' 'medical foods,' or 'food for special dietary use'"(Heller 2005, 169). Manufacturers found significant wiggle room in how they label and market their products via this wide swath of regulatory niches, especially post-2003. This regulatory infrastructure facilitated the explosive growth of the functional food market during the aughts.

At the heart of the debates about managing food and supplement labeling during the 1990s and early aughts was a question of how much knowledge about how a *molecule* or mixture of molecules functioned in the human body was needed before market release. This is a question of legibility, of how an entire epistemic system asks and answers questions about how nature works. For those researching and promoting functional foods, technology was critical to making molecules legible, to offer at least some claims that linked structure with function.

Analyzing Antioxidants

Regulatory infrastructures were not the only thing driving researchers, product developers, and marketers to focus in on functional foods. Like Japan, lawmakers and researchers in the United States shared an interest in addressing disease caused by lifestyle and aging. This is most evident in the work of centers and institutes gathered under the umbrella of the US National Institute of Health, especially the National Institute on Aging (NIA). Established in 1974 by an act of Congress, by 1993 the NIA began focusing on translational research that offered to make the findings of basic and clinic-based research applicable to improving life. In other words, they sought to "mainstream the 'bench to bedside'" approach to research and to "[explore] the underlying molecular mechanisms responsible for the functional decline that occurs with aging" while testing interventions into the aging process (National Institute of Health 2017). If familiar molecules such as vitamins E and C, readily available from foods, could help reduce the rate of oxidation in laboratory and animal tests, what other molecules might be out there, and what role might they play?

Understanding the biochemical activity of molecules in the body is the core goal of nutrition research. In 1993, NIA researchers Guouhua Cao, Helaine M. Alessio, and Richard G. Culture published a paper in the journal *Free Radical Biology and Medicine*. Entitled "Oxygen-radical Absorbance Capacity Assay for

Antioxidants," the paper recounts what the authors term a "relatively simple but sensitive and reliable method of quantitating the oxygen-radical absorbing capacity of antioxidants in [blood] serum" (Cao et al. 1993, 303). The paper came at a time when scholarly attention to the role of free radicals—reactive oxygen species—in human diseases had notably increased. Researchers understood that the presence of certain biological molecules, for example, Low Density Lipoprotein (LDL; a form of cholesterol) was linked to increased risk of disease. What they didn't understand was how those molecules acted to cause disease in the body, for example, how elevated levels of LDL might contribute to the formation of atherosclerotic plaques (Jürgens et al. 1987). For researchers in the mid-1990s interested in heart disease, for example, oxidation—a chemical change that occurs when one molecule loses electrons—repeatedly appeared in *in vitro* (aka test tube) laboratory tests as a potential cause of transforming LDL from a relatively benign compound into one that could harm health (Steinberg 1995).[1] This "oxidative modification hypothesis," that modification of the molecular structure of LDL (or other fatty proteins found in blood) via oxidation was core to the development of atherosclerosis, suggested that a specific set of molecular interactions resulted in the transition from health to sickness. It followed, then, that if one could intervene in that specific set of molecular interactions (oxidation), one could possibly delay or prevent disease onset.

Researchers understood a range of compounds as potential sources of oxidative stress. Environmental pollutants, ultraviolet light, or rancid fats all presented the capability of introducing reactive oxygen species into the body. These are molecules that can not only modify proteins, they can also damage DNA. A logical step for those trained in the central tenets of molecular biology, where structure and function are always intertwined, was to investigate whether one could intervene in unwanted damage from reactive oxygen species that bodies encountered in their everyday environment via antioxidants.

Antioxidants are exactly what they sound like: molecules that act against oxidation. In a 1936 patent application, Henry Mattill and Harold Olcott, employees of Lever Brothers (the precursor to Unilever), referred to antioxidants as "inhibitols," molecules with antioxidant "character capable of being used without harmful adulteration of the food substance to be preserved against injurious oxidation changes" (Mattill and Olcott 1937). A familiar example of antioxidants is beta-carotene (water-soluble vitamin A), as well as vitamins C and E. Purified forms of these plant-derived substances have been in use since the 1930s in industrial food production, as additives that prevent rancidity and extend shelf life. As such, it was not much of a leap to go from additives that helped prolong a food's shelf life to molecular ingestibles that could act as inhibitols in the body proper.

Demonstrating the ability of something to inhibit oxidation, however, was less straightforward than researchers would have preferred. Cao, Alessio, and Culture's paper promised otherwise. Although the reported method didn't allow measurement of an individual antioxidant's activity, it did allow evaluation of the *total* antioxidant capacity of serum, and did so in a quantitatively reproducible manner.[2] This meant that researchers could test whether supplementation or diet modification increased the overall amount of antioxidants found in the bloodstream. The assay's ability to quantify the reaction over time, a later review would report, proved especially useful for measuring antioxidant activity found in samples that did not immediately react (Huang et al. 2005, 1846). Cao's method decreased the barrier to demonstrating antioxidant activity. Although not the first, nor only method developed for in vitro measurement of antioxidant levels, the ORAC assay was rapidly improved and widely adopted, notably by Cao's colleagues at the NIA in the National Institute of Health.

Contemporary scientific processes of knowing, as a range of scholars of science and technology note, depend on creating knowledge that can circulate away from the bodies and places where it is produced (Harding 1986; Knorr Cetina 1999; Porter 1996). Reproducible generation of quantitative measures greases the mechanisms of knowledge production. Cao, Alessio, and Culture's method, in creating a mode for quantifying the total presence of antioxidants in serum, offered new possibilities for those researching the role of dietary compounds in increasing antioxidant levels in blood serum, as well as the potential role of these compounds in preventing attacks from reactive oxidative species.

Communicating Molecular Materiality

Between 1993 and 1995, publications about the antioxidant capacity of foods remained relatively constant. However, in 1995, Cao alongside a group of other researchers at the Jean Meyer USDA Human Nutrition Research Center on Aging developed a way of automating the ORAC assay. This drastically decreased the cost of sampling and increased the number of samples that could be tested in a given time (Cao et al. 1995). In line with common nutritional understanding of diet as key to health, and fruits and vegetables as good-for-you foods, researchers at the Center on Aging (and elsewhere) began testing the total antioxidant capacity of a range of foods.

By measuring total antioxidant capacity of foods, the ORAC assay allowed researchers to begin what could be described as an ongoing series of "trials of strength" (Latour 1993, 79), tests that pitted different foods against each other with the goal of revealing which ones might be most applicable in the search to improve and extend human life. Researchers at the Research Center on Aging, led by Cornell-trained researcher Ronald Prior, quickly took advantage of the test's ability to rapidly compare antioxidant capacity of different foods. They started with familiar foods: one of the first and most widely cited of these tests examined the antioxidant capacity of twelve fruits readily available in Boston supermarkets in the winter. Of the twelve fruits tested—(listed here in order of their antioxidant capacity) strawberry, kiwi, plum, orange, red grape, kiwi fruit, pink grapefruit, white grape, banana, apple, tomato, pear, and honeydew—strawberry came out on top, its juice extract two times more effective at preventing oxidation in the assay than orange juice, and greater than thirteen times more effective than honeydew (Wang et al. 1996). Their research demonstrated that the one known antioxidant present in many of these foods—vitamin C—was not the only compound exhibiting antioxidant capacity. This indicated that fruits and vegetables contained additional compounds beyond the familiar vitamins and minerals identified during the first half of the twentieth century that may help prevent oxidation. Later that year, the researchers moved on to vegetables. In a trial of strength between twenty-two vegetables easily found at Boston supermarkets, garlic, kale, spinach, Brussels sprouts, alfalfa sprouts, broccoli florets, and beets performed best (Cao et al. 1996). Viewed through the lens of antioxidant capacity, some fruit and vegetable extracts were distinctly better than others.

Although these trials of strength initially examined fruits and vegetables "local" to the continental United States, researchers soon expanded their efforts to include foodstuffs from more distant locales. The 1996 assay of twenty-two vegetables also examined green and black tea, showing them significantly more effective than any of the vegetables in preventing oxidation *in vitro* against one of the reactive agents (Cao et al. 1996). In placing fruits, vegetables, and a common plant-based beverage in an *in vitro* arena and pitting them against known oxidative stressors, the researchers sought to make visible the micro-contests they hypothesized as occurring in the eating, breathing, aging body.

Building on their findings that fruits and vegetables contained compounds that acted as antioxidants, Prior and colleagues began investigating what chemical structures beyond vitamin C might contribute to antioxidant function

(Cao 1997). In this they followed the logics of nutritional reductionism *and* the core logic of molecular biology: that a molecule's structure shaped its biological function. Moving from total antioxidant capacity, which revealed the entirety of a foodstuff's antioxidant potential, to the particular relationship between a molecule's structure and its function engaged researchers in a process of "molecular imagination" (Landecker 2011, 185). For Hannah Landecker, writing about genetically modified organisms, molecular imagination is a process of "imaginative acts of thinking, visualizing and controlling food" as an external molecular source that can "interact with our internal molecules," and in doing so dissolves the boundaries between one's particular body and the larger landscape that produces the foods we eat (Landecker 2011, 185). Building on knowledge about the molecular structure of known antioxidants such as beta-carotene, researchers focused their attention on specific sub-groups of phytochemicals found in plants: flavonoids and anthocyanins. Isolated, these compounds could be tested and ranked for their antioxidant activity (Wang et al. 1997), and in the process activate new forms of molecular imagination on how plants acted.

Drawing on their understanding of the molecular structure of known antioxidants, researchers began to look more closely at flavonoids and anthocyanins, compounds that contribute to the bright colors in plants (reviewed in Pietta 2000). Identifying these molecules not only as responsible for the vivid color of blueberries or mangos, but also as core players in the antioxidant potential of foods offered a short-cut for communicating with the public about how to identify antioxidant-rich foods. All one needed to do was "eat the rainbow." By 1999, the phrase "Eat the Rainbow" began regularly appearing in mass media outlets, and in 2000 had trickled down enough that a young science fair contestant in Canada took home laurels for her "Eat the Rainbow" project (Jackson 2000). The focus on flavonoids and anthocyanins as the molecular sources of antioxidant activity in whole foods joined an easily accessible visual indicator, color, to the molecularly elucidated ties between molecular structure and *in vitro* (as well as anticipated *in vivo*) function.

The rapid ability to test antioxidant capacity, and resulting ORAC values, facilitated the emergence of new, increasingly molecularized, hierarchies of nutritional value. The ORAC assay not only permitted comparison between strawberries and apples, it also permitted researchers to quantify differences in antioxidant levels *within* plant species (Ehlenfeldt and Prior 2001) and between domesticated and wild cultivars (Deighton et al. 2000). Via the ORAC assay, researchers were also able to enter into conversations about terroir, demonstrating that geographic origin and harvest time could contribute to total antioxidant capacity (Ou et al. 2002).[3] ORAC made the micromolecular components of foods, and their potential interactions with a range of environments, accessible. In addition, the ORAC test (along with other tests of oxidative capacity) closely linked specific molecules and molecular families with their potential to fight off oxidation outside of the test tube, and did so in a way that tied health not only to how people eat, but also to how they considered the entire agricultural process.

Molecular Politics

Despite the significant attention from researchers interested in how food and the body interact, information about antioxidant potential remained scattered in scientific papers rather than publicly aggregated. That changed in 2007 when the USDA released a database listing antioxidant activity as measured by the ORAC procedure for 277 foods. The database compiled a wide range of non-processed and processed foods such as fruits, vegetables, and nuts with more processed foods such as oils, rolled grains, and juices. In 2010, an additional forty-nine foods were added to the database. The authors of the introduction to the 2010 release highlighted that the second version included the addition of maple syrup, açaí, and goji berries (Haytowitz and Bhagwat 2010, i); all three products had gained recent power on the market and carried links to either indigenous foodways or far-flung places of production. The database itself was compiled from data generated by a range of sources. These ranged from foods analyzed by the USDA as part of the National Food and Nutrient Analysis Program, foods collected and analyzed as part of the food composition database for American Indians and Alaskan Natives, data collected from available literature, and data from some food industry sources (Haytowitz and Bhagwat 2010, 2). In other words, the database assembled together and contained a range of different interests.

Although the database highlighted differences in the quality of the data, its true charisma lay in the column containing the results of the varied trials of strength assembled by the database. Those charismatic numbers conveniently assembled by the USDA were easy to extract, reproduce, and repackage into infographics that quickly communicated how potent a food's antioxidant capacity was. For example, the Wild Blueberry Association of North America circulated a press release on May 5, 2008, titled "Blueberry Juice Tops the ORAC Antioxidant Chart." The chart demonstrated the superior antioxidant value of blueberry juice to other juices, using the USDA's own database to bolster the agricultural association's efforts to sell blueberries not just as a fruit, but rather as a value-added juice, a "concentrated sources of protective natural compounds" (Wild Blueberry Association of North America 2008). Once translated into easily digestible graphs, information about antioxidant levels became much more amenable to the print, web-based, and on-package mediums of late twentieth- and early twenty-first-century health communication so critical to efforts to expand consumption in an otherwise inelastic market. The ORAC numbers, assembled together by the USDA website, created a new legibility for a scientific concept—oxidation and its prevention—that otherwise remained relatively resistant to everyday discourse.

The numbers added for the second release of the database carried a different sort of charisma—one that drew on a desire for foods from indigenous or distant sources as evidenced through the inclusion of foodstuffs such as açaí, gogi berry, and mangosteen (McDonell 2016)—a charisma that facilitated extractionist logics. As scholars like Hiʻilei Hobart show in their examination of poi in Hawaiʻi, historic modes of extracting indigenous foods have often relied on use of technology to transform foods from abject to acceptable (2017; see also García 2013). Similarly, measurement of ORAC activities offered the possibility of technologically transforming local food knowledge, geographically situated away from the ills of the "Global North," into products that could be extracted from their whole food milieu and then tested. The resulting trials of strength produced numbers that justified further investment in, and subsequent extraction of, those foods from their agricultural places of production and into the global food market.

In compiling and making public the ORAC database, the USDA as an institution, and its associated researchers, found themselves tangled in an accumulation of interests facilitated by the presence of a collated, government-sponsored database. Like the Wild Blueberry Association, many food producers, importers, marketers, and bloggers found the numbers generated by ORAC assays useful modes for comparing and communicating about foods. The loosened regulatory landscape highlighted above facilitated a proliferation of messaging about products. Packaging and nutrition articles promoted the idea that certain foods contained higher levels of biologically active molecules than others, often represented through graphs comparing ORAC numbers. Others simply invited eaters to activate their imagination of what was happening in the body. Naked's Pomegranate Blueberry juice, for example, noted that "Fresh, pure; If antioxidants are the foot soldiers in the war against cell-damaging free

radicals, then Naked Juice Pomegranate Blueberry is a Five-Star General ....
prepare for battle, drink your super juice and left, right, left your way to good
health" (Table 4.1).[4] Although not explicitly medicinal, communication about
these foods winked and nodded toward larger societal fears about aging and
exposure to the miasmatic dangers of the late twentieth and early twenty-first

Table 4.1 Functional drinks examined, 2009. I have attempted to maintain first
letter formatting in all names and claims

Drink	Flavor	Claims	Messages
Glacéau Vitamin Water	XXX (triple antioxidants) açaí-blueberry-pomegranate	10 calories, antioxidants, vitamins, superfruits, fight free radicals, naturally sweetened	Nutrient rich, calorie poor
SoBe Lifewater	Yumberry Pomegranate Vitamin-Enhanced Water Beverage Purify	Vitamins, herbal content: ginger and dandelion, 0 calories	Purify, life
Purity Organic Water	Orange Mango Water	Electrolytes, 60 calories, organic	Purity, restore, organic
Ayela's Herbal Water	Cloves Cardamom Cinnamon	Zero calories, zero artificial, zero preservatives, organic	Purified water, organic
Penta	Ultra-Purified, Antioxidant Water	Pure antioxidant, neutralizes free radicals, no additives, fully absorbed	Feel more energized and alert today, and healthier for years to come, purity
Sonu Water	Blueberry Pear	Electrolytes, vitamins	Organic
Metromint	Orangemint Water	real mint unsweetened	All natural, pure, relieves your thirst, soothes your body, and revives your soul
Honest Ade	Orange Mango with Mangosteen, Just a Tad Sweet	Less sugar, full day's vitamin C, antioxidant-rich	Purified water, organic
Honest Tea	Pomegranate Red Tea with Goji Berry	Antioxidant power	Purified water, great taste, good health, social impact, heavenly, organic

Drink	Flavor	Claims	Messages
Carpe Diem Kombucha			Cleanses and refreshes your body, your soul, metabolism enhancer, harmonizing effects on metabolism and digestive system, supports the body's immune system; historical precedent of Zen masters, organic
Function: Nightlife	Passionfruit Guava	All Natural, no preservatives, plant extracts and amino acids to support healthy dopamine levels; epimedium, niacin and cnidium get your blood flowing and amp up your stamina; includes a graphical representation of "relative functional units" of each functional ingredient	Helps promote sexual health, support desire, reward, satisfaction and proper circulation; created by physicians
Naked Antioxidant	Pomegranate Blueberry	Antioxidant, 100 percent juice, no added sugar, no preservatives, no inhibitions	Fresh, pure; if antioxidants are the foot soldiers in the war against cell-damaging free radicals, then Naked Juice Pomegranate Blueberry is a Five-Star General .... Prepare for battle, drink your super juice, and left, right, left your way to good health
Bolthouse Farms Heart Healthy	Pear Merlot	Promotes a healthy heart with barliv, 100 percent natural, omega-3-fatty acids, no preservatives, no artificial colors, no artificial flavors, no genetically modified ingredients, antioxidant rich	Heart healthy (FDA approved health claim), organic
Sambazon Açaí Antioxidant Superfood	Supergreens Revolution	2x the antioxidants of blueberries, healthy omegas 3-6-9, delivers phytonutrients, fiber, protein	Pure energy, incredible nutrition, superhealthy, organic

centuries (e.g., Liboiron 2013). In doing so, marketers sought to capture taste buds as well as the larger imagination of how bodies, at the molecular level, engage with environment.

In June 2012, the USDA responded to the exuberant excess of claims-making by withdrawing the database. The USDA's withdrawal revealed an ongoing molecular politics where *how* one understands a food's efficacy shapes *how* one orders and regulates knowledge. USDA researchers at the Human Nutrition Research Center on Aging had been tasked from the very get-go to develop translational research, to make the leap from *in vitro* findings to *in vivo* experimentation[5] with the aim of making life better. As such, a logic of extraction sat at the very core of their efforts. In withdrawing the database, the USDA sought to remove the appearance of any institutional belief in the capability of *in vitro* antioxidative assays to demonstrate the efficacy of natural or processed foods in intervening in *in vivo* processes. Labels, magazine articles, blog posts, and the like followed suit, moving away from presenting ORAC numbers and toward other modes of communication. The fad, one might assume, had peaked.

From ORAC to Superfoods

Even as functional foods faded into an everyday part of the US grocery store landscape, the subsequent success of superfoods as a communication category, when read within the framing of extractionist logics, suggests that the discovery and characterization of antioxidants were not simply a fad. Searching for a better life at the end of the twentieth century calls into being a certain form of individual: one equipped with the skillset to live and eat in ways that promote health. It calls for extraction of knowledge about the goodness of various foods, and molecules, in caring for the body (cf. Ives, this volume). Rather than ORAC assays doing the work of extracting the antioxidant value of various foods, it is now individual brains that are invited to do the work of looking at something and extrapolating whether the food will contain biologically active molecules.

Although the move to superfoods superficially appears to repudiate molecular extraction via technology as a mode of attaining health (recall the Whole Foods focus on "wholeness" mentioned above), the molecular continues to play a core role in communication. Even as use of ORAC numbers dropped, marketers, nutrition writers, and bloggers continued to mobilize a molecular understanding of whole fruits and vegetables as carriers of health-promoting molecules. They did so by drawing on the relationships between antioxidant activity and color.

The idea that color could act as a short-cut to understanding the molecular content of plants without the work of going through a laboratory easily entered into the mass communication infrastructures of the early twenty-first century. Dynamic, colorful infographics urging children and adults to "Eat the Rainbow" have proliferated from public and private sources. Many still link the colors of the rainbow as found in fruits and vegetables to specific families of molecules and specific sorts of health-promoting properties. Swissotel, for example, has drawn together a chart using data from thirty-two public research institutions and privately owned health reporting resources that highlights how "**Red** foods contain phytochemicals including lycopene and anthocyanins ... **Orange|Yellow** foods are packed with carotenoids ... and tend to contain an abundance of vitamins and fibre ... Chlorophyll, the pigment that makes plants **green**, is loaded with antioxidants ... **Blue|Purple** loaded with anthocyanins and resveratrol ... **White** coloured by anthoxanthins, they might also contain the beneficial phytonutrients allicin and quercetin" ("Colorful Foods: The Benefits of Eating the Rainbow" 2017). Although no longer linked to their specific ORAC values, the understanding of these pigmented molecules as potent antioxidants remains an easily legible bridge between the extracted fortification of functional foods and the wholeness of superfoods. Similarly, the healthy nature of colorful foods easily entered into the super-saturated, digitally perfected space of online platforms and apps. As a glance at the over 6 million #superfood- or #superfoods-tagged posts on Instagram shows, naturally occurring colors continue to mark a food's micronutrient and health-promoting status. Color as a marker of health corresponds especially well with the short-cut visuality of social media, allowing content generators and content consumers to quickly communicate about the health of an item and, in the process, signal their own stance on health maintenance (cf. Sikka 2019). Although the explicit technological engagement that characterized (and characterizes) functional food advertising is less apparent, technological extraction remains, haunting the images through the linkage between color and health that has now become common knowledge.

While infographics may highlight whole foods, it is notable that many (although not all—quinoa and rooibos offer notable counterpoints) of the foods promoted as superfoods are also significantly processed. As LeBlanc, Guthman, and Brondizio highlight in this volume, powdered smoothie mixes, juices, and energy bars make up a significant set of the industrial superfood market. These items, like their functional food counterparts, similarly offer to extract the powerful nutritive properties from food on behalf of consumers. The core difference between the two categories, rather, shows up in how explicitly extractionist logics are mobilized: marketing of functional foods specifically draws on scientific research to make its claims, while marketing of superfoods relies rather on the ability of a vague technological understanding, developed during the 1990s and early aughts, to facilitate translation between color, general molecular category, and health.

Ideas, Extracted

Extractionist logics function by linking together scientific research and technological innovation with the creation of an activated imagination of how molecules behave. The work of creating this mass molecular imagination does not just lie in the realm of nutritionists or marketers. Rather, the creation of a wide-ranging understanding of certain groups of molecules as having positive, disease-fighting impact on bodies comes into being via the action of a wide range of actors and interests. Research into the biological ability of molecules to prevent oxidation facilitated extractionist logics by enabling rapid, cost-effective screening of the antioxidant activity of a range of foodstuffs. Published antioxidant activity levels, embodied in the ORAC score, became communication devices that marketers and others used to compare familiar and unfamiliar products. These entered into already existing infrastructures, from the trade groups discussed elsewhere in this volume (Reisman) to the desires for foods that reconnected one to nature.

Distributed between researchers, policymakers, food producers, food marketers, and eaters, extractionist logics propose that the most valuable parts of foods—their micromolecular structures, found in microbial metabolites or the colorful phytochemicals fabricated through the plant-based labor of growing and reproducing—are there to be extracted, isolated, and reproduced through scientific and technological innovation. Once re-embodied in functional foods, these molecules and their accompanying logics situate eaters as micro-extractors, capable of using the knowledge they have gained through immersion in a saturated media environment to responsibly navigate and extract extra health-promoting value via consumption choices. Herein lies the continuum between functional and superfoods: both build on an epistemic foundation of examining antioxidant activity that has been used to create, excite, and profit from a molecular imagination informed by techno-science. Superfoods, like functional foods, are valued because they carry the potential of intervening in long-term human health. And, like functional foods, they remain epistemic objects that resist complete characterization.

Notes

1   Steinberg, who founded the University of California, San Diego's School of Medicine, is credited with the development of the oxidation hypothesis/oxidative modification hypothesis. Building on work that began in 1979 examining how macrophages were metabolized in cell culture, Steinberg's research career focused on understanding the biochemical mechanisms that led to the creation of atherosclerotic lesions. For a retrospective of his life's work see Steinberg (2009).

2   They did this by taking advantage of the fluorescent properties of an indicator protein. When oxidated, the level of fluorescence changes. The ability to detect this change and plot it out on a graph allowed researchers to quantify the reaction rate, and in the process quantify the effectiveness of antioxidants added to the serum.

3   It should be noted that the study by Ou et al., which examined an astonishing 927 samples, came out of Brunswick Laboratories. The group helped commercialize the ORAC assay.

4   All drinks but the Vitamin Water and Sobe Lifewater were purchased from Whole Foods in New York City; drinks were selected based on category of functional drink (enhanced water, tea, smoothie, other) and location within the refrigerated drink wall—all drinks were spatially separated from the "bottled water" section. Vitamin Water was obtained from a ten-day promotional event held at 626 Broadway during early April 2009; Sobe Lifewater was purchased at Key Foods. I chose Whole Foods as the primary purchase site due to the significant selection of functional beverages available in their refrigerated drinks section. I excluded sports and energy drinks from this survey based on the definition of functional drinks as offering some health benefit beyond that of basic nutrition.

5   Researchers found that consuming fruits and veggies raised the antioxidative capability of blood serum when that serum was tested using the ORAC assay. Such findings don't necessarily mean long-term health, of course, a tricky proposition given the nuance of food consumption versus the blunt force of pharmaceuticals.

Part Two

Working Miracles

"A Really Good Story Behind It": Moringa Bars and Venture Capital Funding

Julie Guthman

In 2016, I attended an event in San Francisco, billed as an opportunity for "disruptive" food start-ups to connect with interested venture capitalists. Agriculture and food have become the newest domains of Silicon Valley investment, animated only in part by the foodie culture that pervades the region but more so by a commonly held view in the valley that agriculture and food are under-invested and therefore ripe for Silicon Valley-style innovation. This particular event, dubbed "FoodBytes," was a "pitch" event, mainly involving hubristic entrepreneurs attempting to attract venture capital funding for products that they claimed would solve major problems in the food system.

In addition to the requisite on-stage pitches were the product displays. Many consisted of cookies and nutritional bars made of newly discovered superfoods or unusual ingredients such as crickets, which were touted for their abilities to address problems such as malnutrition or global climate change and sometimes both. Pondering how bars in convenient packaging would be received and utilized by the malnourished in the developing world, I was reminded of tech critic Evgeny Morozov's critique of solutionism. For Morozov (2013), "solutionism" is "an intellectual pathology that recognizes problems as problems based on just one criterion: whether they are solvable with a nice and clean technological solution at our disposal." With its inattention to the actual causes of any given problem, solutionism had run amok at this event and continues to pervade the tech world writ large, where the designers of many products seem to be in search of problems that their innovations can solve.

Not exactly so for one of the featured bars at this event. This one caught my eye because it had a somewhat different story behind it. It was made from the leaves of the moringa tree, *Moringa oleifera*, commonly referred to as either the drumstick tree or horseradish tree. *Moringa oleifera* is thought to be native to India but has been widely introduced and naturalized across the tropics and subtropics, to the extent that it is classified as an invasive species. Its invasiveness may owe to its resiliency; it can grow in poor soil, and in extremely hot and dry climates (Paynter 2018), therefore making it a good candidate for "climate-smart" agriculture. In addition, it has many uses, including as a scent stabilizer in cosmetics, a means of water purification, a cooking oil, animal fodder, and a nitrogen-fixing mulch. Still, it is perhaps most noted and valued for what the leaves provide to humans, whether in salads, soups, teas, or traditional medical preparations. Unusually, the leaves consist of 15–20 percent protein and are inclusive of all nine essential amino acids. In addition, they are rich in various micronutrients, including vitamins C and D, as well as potassium, iron, and calcium (CABI 2019; Kuli Kuli 2019; Paratore 2013). Like quinoa, moringa has qualities of both a "miracle food" and a "miracle crop," with capacity to address problems from world hunger to climate change (McDonell 2015) (see also McDonell, Brondizio, this volume for other examples of multifunctional crops). Rather than a product of design, in other words, moringa stands as an example of a found, not made, solution—and one that might address multiple problems.

At the event, the start-up company Kuli Kuli was promoting moringa and handing out samples of snack bars made from the leaves. It soon became clear that Kuli Kuli bars were not destined for the malnourished in the developing world but for busy US consumers seeking to improve their health and wellbeing. In her pitch, Lisa Curtis, the company's CEO and co-founder, articulated her aim to address "a market hungry for superfood here in the US," touting moringa as "the new kale." Since moringa would not be marketed as fresh greens, she made what have become *de rigueur* nods to convenience, claiming the company would "make it easy for Americans to get their greens on the go," providing "a salad in a bar" because Americans "want to increase their servings of vegetables but they don't always have time to eat a salad." At the same time, she noted that her overall vision was to help improve nutrition and livelihoods worldwide. To that end, the company was working with women's cooperatives throughout the developing world to source the moringa, aspiring to provide them with enhanced economic opportunities.[1] In addition, it was "using our supply chain to help re-forest a country." Here Curtis was referring to their efforts in Haiti—"for any of you who have heard of Haiti"—where, in partnership with Whole Foods and the Clinton Foundation, the company was planting moringa trees to make profitable opportunities for the people there, as well. Curtis then called out for "mission-aligned investors" who were interested in "nourishing you and nourishing the world." After noting that standing out (among investors) comes down to telling a story, she capped her five-minute pitch with "we want it to taste good, we want it to be good for the world, and we want it to have a really good story behind it." Hers was a masterful pitch, and pitches are apparently critical for obtaining start-up funding (Goldstein 2018).

In this chapter, I bring attention to the site of *investment* for superfoods. Superfoods not only need markets, they need funding, and attracting investment capital is a unique craft, especially in the tech-saturated world of Silicon Valley in which Kuli Kuli has positioned itself. Here I draw on Goldstein's incisive examination of entrepreneur-funder relations in the "clean tech space," to note how funders insist on both world-changing vision (a.k.a. "disruption") and capital discipline. Regarding the latter, to be funded entrepreneurs must display their willingness to succumb to the dictates of marketability, cost efficiency, and, hence, profitability. A focus on investment therefore sheds light on an under-examined dimension of Silicon Valley-type solutionism—and that is the need to have a sellable commodity by which profits can be made sooner than later. It is only with a viable "plan to market" that both entrepreneurs and venture capitalists can get their "exits," referring to buy-outs by larger companies. Superfood products lend themselves to this kind of solutionism because they are easily reformulated and made into what the industry refers to as "consumer packaged goods." As such, they render socioenvironmental problems less technical (cf. Li 2007) than commodifiable.[2]

I thus take a closer look at the "really good story behind it," gleaned from online articles about Curtis and the company, in addition to the pitch she made that day. These sources illustrate how her attempts to bridge development aspirations, nutritional improvement through superfoods, and doing well by doing good have attracted significant attention by funders and others. This is in part because in the world of venture capital the story is the initial commodity, the basis by which entrepreneurs get their first cash infusions and sometimes their exits, and her story excites on many fronts. At the same time, the win-win-win articulated in Curtis's approach is not so easily achieved, especially with a business model founded in export-oriented developmentalism, nutritionism, and social entrepreneurism, all of which have also been subject to scholarly critique for their perverse consequences. As such, the decisions she has made and may well make in the future will nearly certainly deliver less than her initial vision. They nevertheless reveal her willingness to be disciplined by capital, the other requisite piece of obtaining funding. The divergence between what sells to venture capital and what can actually do good is one of the ways that "green capital"-funded efforts in the tech sector end up with low-hanging fruit (Goldstein 2018, 139), such that little progress is made, with the potential to foreclose more serious solutions to deeply rooted problems.

The Company Story

A graduate of Whitman College in Washington state, where she had served as the sustainability coordinator, Lisa Curtis had built an impressive résumé before she became the founder of Kuli Kuli. She had interned at the White House, represented North American youth at the United Nations Environment Programme, served as an impact investment project assistant for Startup India, a communications director at a solar energy company, and a freelance writer for *Forbes* and the *Huffington Post* (Curtis 2019). Yet it was her experience in the Peace Corps that was the basis of the story of Kuli Kuli.

Curtis was doing her Peace Corps stint in Niger in 2010–11, when she began to feel quite tired and weak. She surmised that as a vegetarian she may have been lacking sufficient protein in her diet, given what was available at the local markets. In one version of the story her mom had been shipping her energy bars. One day, she and a woman from the village had come across a malnourished child. The woman then suggested to Curtis that she bring the child some *"kuli* bars*"* referring to the energy bars Curtis kept around (Laskow 2014). Most versions of the story are somewhat more compelling. They tell how women in the village introduced Curtis to the leaves of the moringa tree to address her physical weakness. The leaves were wrapped in a peanut paste called *kuli-kuli*, eaten by the Hausa people of West Africa (Paratore 2013; Tsai 2013). As Curtis began to feel better, she went looking for more *kuli-kuli*. A woman who was able to understand her broken Hausa gave her an entire sack of *kuli-kuli* and refused to let her pay for it. Among other things, the experience of having a total stranger give her food in one of the most malnourished countries in the world stuck with her (Paratore 2013). So did the experience of recovering her energy from something other than her *"kuli"* from home.

Having directly experienced the benefits of this miracle plant, Curtis started to think about promoting it in Niger, somewhat begging the question of why malnourished people were not already eating it. This plan was quickly shunted aside following the kidnapping of two French men, allegedly by members of Al Qaeda, after which the Peace Corps suspended its program in Niger (Laskow 2014). Forced to leave the country seven months after her arrival, Curtis relocated to India to take part in an impact investment program, where she learned about the world of start-ups (Curtis 2019; Laskow 2014).

But moringa kept nagging at her. So, in May 2013, she "partnered" with some childhood friends to form the company Kuli Kuli and opted to base it in Oakland, California. After having considered tea, pesto, and hummus made from moringa leaves as their products, they opted to go with bars. With its sort of "green taste," allegedly similar to matcha, much of what would go in the bar to make it palatable would be nuts, dates, other fruit, agave, or chocolate (Laskow 2014; Tsai 2013). The company then located a co-manufacturer in Washington State to produce the prototype bars they had in mind. The company had hoped to use local Bay Area labor, but the manufacturers in the Bay Area all required high minimum runs. Naturally, the company also sought funding. Thanks to the JOBS Act of 2012, a law that eased many US securities laws, the company was able to utilize a crowd-financing mechanism (Laskow 2014). They went to IndieGoGo, a crowd-funding platform for entrepreneurs, and raised $53,000. With funding and a manufacturing facility, and a lot of pavement-pounding, Curtis was able to get some Whole Foods outlets to feature her bars (Feldman 2017; Paratore 2013; Tsai 2013).

It was apparently never an option to hand out these moringa bars in the country of origin. In Niger, Curtis had watched USAID pull up every week with flag-stamped American corn and was aware of research showing how food aid can be detrimental to agricultural development. She concluded that the better approach would be to "empower" women to grow and sell it (Laskow 2014; Tsai 2013). "We want every woman in West Africa to have a *Moringa oleifera* tree in her yard and the knowledge to harness its nutrients," she stated in an interview. She quoted the old adage about giving a man a fish and he'd eat for a day while teaching him to fish would allow him to eat for the rest of his life (quoted in Paratore 2013). She set out to improve women's livelihoods by enrolling them in the market.

Obtaining the moringa was challenging, though. The tree's leaves are delicate. If not boiled (the traditional preparation), they need to be washed and ground into a powder within an hour or two of plucking to prevent rot (Paynter 2018). Curtis had hoped to work with women in Niger to obtain the moringa but found it difficult and costly to have it prepared and shipped from a landlocked country. Plus, she found that not that many groups in Niger were producing it. She then learned of a women's group in Ghana that was trying to export moringa and began working with them instead (Feldman 2017). Later she extended the network of producers to women's grower cooperatives elsewhere, with most coming from Ghana, involving about 500 women (Feldman 2017; Paratore 2013; Tsai 2013). She told one source that she hoped she would eventually obtain and sell all that these women could supply (Tsai 2013), but in other interviews Curtis was more measured. A different source reported that in addition to importing moringa Curtis was "partnering" with local organizations to increase local consumption of the leaves, and therefore was not sourcing too much from any one organization (Paratore 2013).

With more suppliers, Kuli Kuli needed more capital. This time the company went to another crowd-funding mechanism: Ag Funder, making it the first company to raise both start-up and first round investment capital with such mechanisms (Laskow 2014). By 2017, the company had raised a total of $4.25 million in additional capital, including financing from Kellogg's venture capital arm, Eighteen94 Capital, and other institutional investors such as InvestEco and S2G Ventures (Burwood-Taylor 2017). The company was backed also by philanthropic investors including the Clinton Foundation (Waite 2018). By 2018, Kuli Kuli had expanded the product line to include powders and shots, was being marketed in Target, Safeway, Albertsons, Costco, CVS, as well as Whole Foods, and had expanded its grower network to Haiti, Nicaragua, and thirteen other developing countries (Feldman 2017; Paynter 2018). Curtis had even been granted federal funds. In August 2018, Kuli Kuli received a federal grant from the Millennium Challenge Corporation, a foreign aid agency that focuses on helping countries fight terrorism by fighting poverty. This particular grant brought the company back to Niger, one of the targets of the Corporation's anti-terrorist activities. The grant enabled Kuli Kuli to test the feasibility of having Niger farmers supply moringa (Paynter 2018).

Meanwhile Kuli Kuli incorporated as a bonafide Benefit Corporation (a B Corp), meaning that its obligations would extend beyond its shareholders to include social and environmental benefits. Curtis made this decision before the last round of funding so investors would know Kuli Kuli's aspirations (Feldman 2017). The environmental benefits they would produce included planting trees, often done in collaboration with nonprofits (Paynter 2018). They also began testing for pesticide residues and making sure that their products met organic standards (Feldman 2017).

As a business, however, Kuli Kuli increasingly had to deal with a competitive marketplace. Other purveyors got into the moringa act, often purchasing the material from India where the price was lower. As the company discovered that some moringa labeled as organic had pesticide residues and was more bitter, the company found itself in a position of having to educate consumers not only about the superfood attributes of moringa but about the value of Kuli Kuli the brand, so it could still pay their suppliers a premium (Feldman 2017). So they brought their marketing in-house and hired professionals who could focus on their story. Made possible by the venture capital partnership, they also received technical support from Kellogg's food scientists who helped them formulate a better tasting and more attractive bar (Crawford 2018).

By 2019, Kuli Kuli was poised for even more growth, and one of the avenues of growth was other products, as well as other plants with yet to be revealed qualities. "There are so many plants around the world that Americans don't know," Curtis told one of her interviewers. "We can become a brand that really stands for sustainably-sourced, value added super food products that nourish the communities where they are sourced" (Feldman 2017). The company also began paying more attention to diversity of both the bio and social kind, by asking its suppliers to intercrop moringa with other plants and looking to hire people of color in its Oakland offices (Guest 2019).[3] As for Curtis herself, she had become a darling of the food start-up world, sporting, among other things, a fellowship at Unreasonable, "an organization, investment fund, and private global network dedicated to supporting entrepreneurs positioned to bend history in the right direction" (Curtis 2019).

The success of the company surely does rest on Curtis's story of being healed by moringa with *kuli-kuli* provided by poor women in Niger, having gone on to pay it forward by helping (other) women in the developing world become entrepreneurial moringa exporters, and becoming a smashing social entrepreneur herself by marketing a superfood. Thinking counterfactually, the story simply wouldn't be as compelling if, say, she handed out moringa in its countries of origin, or if consumers weren't willing to eat a superfood in bars. The story of this superfood in that way is indeed a perfect one for attracting venture capital investors, putting development aspirations in a commodity form that will be purchased by well-to-do Americans. The question is whether Kuli Kuli can be as super in actually meeting its multiple goals, especially given the need to turn a profit.

Pillars of the Story

The charm of Curtis's story is in her weaving together doing good, eating well, and doing well monetarily. In less-honeyed terms we might think of her story as bridging export-oriented developmentalism, nutritionism, and social entrepreneurism. But all three of these orientations have been critiqued for providing less than they promise, and it is unclear how Kuli Kuli's approach escapes these critiques, especially with already existing evidence of compromises Curtis has had to make. While the story may work well for attracting funding, it may be much less compelling as a found solution.

Export-oriented Developmentalism

Kuli Kuli's story invites praise for the company's aspirations to develop livelihood opportunities for women in the developing world. Curtis's recognition that hunger cannot be solved by handing out nutritional bars but by giving women an opportunity to produce and sell moringa seems to be informed by Amartya Sen's (1981) ground-breaking entitlement approach. Sen argued vociferously against the notion that hunger and famine result from insufficient food production—or there not being enough food to eat. He posited that hunger results instead from a failure of entitlements—a lack of sufficient means to access food. He noted several ways in which people acquire food beyond growing their own. These include selling a commodity they produce in order to buy food, selling their labor for wages to buy food, or through social means of support, be they inheritance, state assistance, or informal networks. Through an entitlement approach, in short, providing women a market to sell moringa is one of several legitimate means to address hunger.

But is it really? While Curtis's critique of USAID and its history of undercutting farmers is apt (and in keeping with phenomena noted by Sen), she nevertheless reveals her predilections in her repeated references to the allegory about teaching a man to fish. That, along with her reference to women's empowerment and her emphasis on creating export markets for the women, suggests Curtis has been highly persuaded by more recent approaches to economic development that emphasize trade not aid, as well as governmentalities that conflate making entrepreneurial subjects with empowerment.

Following the debt crisis of the 1980s, export-oriented development became the darling of the World Bank, IMF, and other development institutions, which promoted market-oriented solutions—first as debt repayment and then later as poverty alleviation. Many countries encouraged farmers to produce so-called non-traditional exports, crops, and other agricultural products that were of higher value, and sometimes more novel, than those that had underpinned the development of the world food economy in the colonial period (Friedmann 1993; Weis 2007; see also McDonell, this volume). Increasingly such market-oriented approaches were wrapped in the cloak of governmentalities about minimizing dependence and creating entrepreneurial subjects. Through micro-lending, technical aid, and enrollment in business ventures, women, in particular, became the target of "pro-poor" development projects bent on entrepreneurship (Dolan 2012, 2014; Mosse 2013; Rankin 2001; Walker et al. 2008). As Tania Li (2007) has suggested, those championing such schemes were acting in the capacity of trustees, "a position defined by the claim to know how others should live, to know what is best for them, to know what they need" (p. 4).

The problem is that the promise of export-oriented development as an approach to hunger has not borne out empirically. Rather than eliminating dependencies, programs aimed at export-oriented agricultural development made many developing world subjects highly dependent on international markets (Schneider and McMichael 2011). High-value crops are particularly sensitive to price swings or, worse, eventual disinterest in the crop being produced. So, at the very least Kuli Kuli's export-oriented development, while providing cash now, is also subjecting the women entrepreneurs to the whims of a volatile market. Such cash cropping schemes have also in some cases enabled neglect of household food crops, with the potential to worsen hunger (Schroeder 1993). This is not a given, of course, because if moringa earns these women cash they will be able to buy household food—assuming that some producers remain in the business of supplying local markets—or the women grow household crops in addition to moringa. Another issue, if quinoa serves as an appropriate example, is that creating a major export market for moringa has the potential to raise the price of moringa in its indigenous context and in that way contribute to malnutrition (McDonell 2015). Kuli Kuli's press and promotional material do not discuss whether it is a commodity crop in the places from where it hails, or is mainly gathered from backyard gardens and common areas. Yet, it is not clear that export production won't have other consequences for domestic food security, as many schemes have. It is telling that Curtis appears to have backed off her goal to obtain as much moringa as the women could produce, as that would directly undermine her claims about encouraging moringa consumption where it is grown.

What is eminently clear, however, is that Kuli Kuli's vision is not really about teaching the women to fish so they can fish for the rest of their lives. That is an allegory about self-sufficient subsistence production. It is about getting them to sell fish, so they can sell it for the rest of their lives, given the strong potential for declining prices that could increase the precarity of their livelihoods. Having price-taking suppliers in the supply chain may be attractive to venture capital but it seems a far cry from the "empowerment" promised in these approaches.

There is an additional aspect of the Kuli Kuli business model as it relates to the supply chain, illustrated in Curtis's interest in finding other plants besides moringa "that Americans don't know." While bioprospecting has been cast as a way to bring cash to poor economies, in practice most companies have treated native plants and local knowledge about their use as common property ready for the taking, making it an inherently extractive approach rather than one of reciprocity (Shiva 2007). (See also Brondizio, Ives, and McDonell, this volume; cf. Spackman, this volume, who uses extractivism to connote molecularization.) That Kuli Kuli products are being manufactured in the United States rather than in the countries from which moringa is sourced also calls into question the potential of the company to improve incomes in developing economies.

Nutritionism

The traditional method of preparing moringa involves boiling it several times to remove its bitter taste. Doing so, however, drains it of nutrients. For that reason, the Kuli Kuli company has become involved in educational campaigns in moringa growing countries about the nutritional value of the plant and how to prepare it to best take advantage of its nutritional content. Apparently, the "local knowledge" so valuable to the moringa story is deficient and also requires trusteeship (Paynter 2018). While there are nods to expanding moringa consumption in the places where it grows, the business model of Kuli Kuli is based on selling it to US consumers. Kuli Kuli's funding success therefore rests on convincing investors that moringa will be taken seriously as a superfood, desirable and market-worthy enough for consumers to choose it over other nutritional bars, especially given a marketing landscape characterized by abundant competition for snacks (Laskow 2014).

In many ways this isn't difficult. As noted by Crawford (2006), the 1980s saw the rise of "healthism," the notion that health is the highest value, trumping other social concerns. Moreover, this new health consciousness was about more than the absence of illness, but rather about positive steps to optimize one's health (Skrabanek 1994). Optimizing health became an obsession of sorts of the white middle classes especially. A particular bent of healthism arose in the form of what Gyorgy Scrinis (2013) dubbed nutritionism, referring to the framing of food in terms of the role that constituent nutrients and substances play in enhancing human health. The nutritionist call was not about eating your grandmother's chicken soup; it was a call to learn and apply knowledge of the health-promoting aspects of particular nutrients in order to optimize them in one's diet.

With the aid of the public health nutrition community, diet gurus, and food manufacturers themselves, the ideology of nutritionism led to what Scrinis describes as a reductionist approach to nutrition such that obtaining specific nutrients, vitamins, and other constituent elements of food came to take precedence over eating a variety of whole foods. Even though daily vitamins had been around for a while, enhanced supplementation was one manifestation of this. It was imagined that in supplementation the elements deemed to be "good for you" played analogous, if not improved roles in the body as they did when they were found in actual food, and taken in through a meal. It was additionally imagined that bodies, nutrients, and foods were fundamentally similar—that a given thing could have the same effect no matter where and how eaten by whom and that supplementation would not interfere with nutrient absorption of "real" food (Scrinis 2013).

The superfood trend is arguably a newer manifestation of this reductionist approach to nutrition. As defined by Scrinis (2013, 174), superfoods are ordinary whole foods with especially high concentrations of functionally beneficial nutrients. They are elevated by their promise of "wellness," "marketed as though they have medication-grade power to give us stronger and better bodies" (Noble 2018). Unlike dietary supplements, such foods might contain a variety of what Aya Kimura (2013) calls "charismatic" nutrients—those that promise to address specific areas of deficiency rather than just fill the body. Indeed, like quinoa, moringa has no one particular charismatic nutrient (cf. McDonell 2015). Rather it is a food that provides multiple benefits.[4]

Yet, the high-nutrition content of moringa is not a guarantee it will improve the health of its users. That would assume that the bio-available nutrients are not regularly found in people's diets (Scrinis 2013, 175). Maybe not for people in Niger, but is that the case for the yoga pants-wearing classes who are the intended market for Kuli Kuli products?[5] Casting ordinary American diets as insufficient may test plausibility, so the safer route is casting them as not easily had. Indeed, that has been a key feature of what Noble (2018) of the The

Counter aka New Food Economy calls "snackification", one of "several trends that food manufacturers are convinced are the key to their survival." For Noble, "snackification" is a "fixation with convenience rooted in the suspicion that we're all too busy to eat sit-down meals." Kuli Kuli's marketing is in complete concurrence with this model, resting on the presumption that people just don't have time to sit down for a nutritious meal. They could thus use a "salad in a bar" from a "multivitamin in a tree" as Curtis put it (Tsai 2013).

Another aspect of moringa bars is also cause for skepticism on the nutrition front. As we have seen, moringa leaves in their raw form do not travel well; they must be dried and made into powders. These material qualities of moringa must therefore be reformulated into something else if they are to be manufactured elsewhere. At the same time, because moringa doesn't taste very good and is gritty (Tsai 2013), it needs to be disguised to be enjoyed with tasty ingredients—ingredients that may undermine its likeness to salad. Like other superfoods discussed in this volume (see Spackman; LeBlanc, this volume), moringa requires significant reformulation for transport and marketing, at the possible expense of its ultra-nutritional qualities, as well as added ingredients that might make it less healthful. The bar I was handed at the FoodBytes event contains 17 grams of sugar, albeit obtained from dates and tapioca syrup as well as cane sugar. Kuli Kuli bars are thus substantially different than the leaves of the moringa tree wrapped in the peanut paste that inspired the story. At best, then, moringa's superfood status puts a health halo on a food that might otherwise appear just a processed snack (Scrinis 2013, 176).

Social Entrepreneurism

Kuli Kuli, as we have seen, operates under a social enterprise model. The theory for social entrepreneurship and its premise of multiple bottom lines, as put by one of Curtis's observers, is that "when an organization is run as a business rather than a nonprofit, with an eye toward growth, it can do more good in the long run" (see also Alvord et al. 2004; Cho 2006; Day and Steyeart 2012; quoted from Tsai 2013). Lauded by business schools, social enterprise models have been largely dismissed by the Left as another form of corporate greenwashing (Stecker 2016). Writing on the cleantech energy sector, Jesse Goldstein (2018) offers up a more complex analysis. Entrepreneurs want to do good, and indeed are rewarded for their big aspirations by capital markets that want impact. And yet, these same markets discipline what creative innovators can do. Funders want return, and entrepreneurs are not taken too seriously if they put too much emphasis on their good works. This dynamic is readily seen at pitch nights where entrepreneurs almost perfunctorily state their desires to change the world and then get to the real business of articulating their plan to get to market. The key then is walking that fine line—promising an impact greater than making money but showing a willingness to submit to the reins of capital (Goldstein 2018, 62).

Curtis has walked that line carefully, and she has not strayed too far from her mission as she sees it. According to one of her interlocutors, she initially chose crowd-funding to demonstrate that the company had a mission behind it (Laskow 2014). She chose to incorporate as a B Corp to hold herself accountable to the mission. She admits that she didn't originally imagine working with General Mills or Kellogg's "but they brought so much more to the table than capital" in terms of forwarding her mission (Feldman 2017). She has insisted on agricultural practices that are less environmentally deleterious and forged collaborations with nonprofit organizations to plant trees.

And yet, it appears that Curtis is quite willing to be disciplined by capital, and sometimes at the expense of doing good. At least as reported, her decisions have not lost sight of the business side. The trees that Curtis boasts of planting are also there to shore up Kuli Kuli's supply chain, and these efforts at reforestation effectively subsidize her business, just as her testing of pesticide residues to maintain her organic label is driven by making her product stand out. In addition, it should be noted that when Curtis has encountered friction in her social aims, she has turned elsewhere. She dropped her goal of supporting Oakland's local economy when local manufacturers wouldn't provide what she wanted. More pointedly, until that government grant came along, she dropped the idea of sourcing moringa from Niger. Despite that Niger is where she saw such extensive malnourishment so to inspire her effort originally, the women in Niger were ill-positioned to grow enough moringa for Kuli Kuli's needs, and it was too expensive to get it to market. So she replaced them with women from Ghana (as if all African women are interchangeable). And her willingness to work with Kellogg's in reformulating the bar has resulted in a bar that may taste better but contains significant amounts of sugar. More generally Curtis has not been reticent in growing the company, even if that means prospecting for other plants that have little to do with the women of Niger who originally introduced her to moringa, potentially threatening the narrative foundations of the very story that got the company rolling. What, then, really sells Kuli Kuli?

Taken together, several aspects of the Kuli Kuli story have likely been attractive to venture capital. Associating a food with an exotic other has become a useful mode of product differentiation (for example, McDonell 2015). Unlike quinoa, however, this association creates a halo on a particular company and its brand. Unlike other processed bars, Kuli Kuli is also underpinned by neo-development claims. And yet, unlike fair trade chocolate and coffee brands, which do similar work, it is attached to plausible wellness claims. The superfood status of moringa provides a similar halo on the sugar and chocolate present in the bar. In short, to the extent that Kuli Kuli is successful, it is in part because it fruitfully combines a number of qualities that promise to appeal to health-conscious do-gooders. It is like the Whole Foods of snack bars, promising to do good by eating well (cf. Johnston 2008).

Ultimately, though, it may be Curtis herself who underwrites the entire enterprise. Goldstein (2018) notes that once a tech inventor has created a workable model for an idea, venture capitalists want to hand the company over to someone who can manage the business. After all, inventors will want to get the invention right, while business managers will want to get to the business of making money. But Curtis isn't an inventor, and, indeed, what makes Kuli Kuli sellable (to venture capital) is her story and her belief in her story. She believes that she's helping women in the developing world by giving them a market, that she's contributing to consumer health by providing them a superfood that can be eaten on the go, and that she can balance profit-making with social benefit. Moreover, as both a woman and former Peace Corps volunteer, Curtis is better able to play the part of the giver, effectively softening the extractive aspects of the scheme, if not altogether obscuring it. Whether she is doing well by doing good or doing good by doing well, if her new-found visibility and status are any indication, she herself is the embodiment of imagined social entrepreneurism. She has not only mastered the pitch; she is the pitch. Without her ability to sell the win-win-win of her story, all Kuli Kuli offers is another snack bar.

The Problem with the Story

Perhaps, though, the problem is not only that the win-win-win of Kuli Kuli delivers less than it promises. Here it may be useful to view this story through the lens of what Goldstein (2018) refers to as "green capital denial." In using this terminology, he riffs off of Norgaard's (2011) notion of climate change denial. Norgaard's concern is less about denial of the science of climate change, but denial of the reality of what we'd have to do to confront it. Goldstein thus asks if there's another denial going on that is also "planetary in scale, equally abstract, all encompassing, and seemingly unstoppable—that also must immediately be addressed" (p. 141) referring to something no less than capitalism. What he is suggesting is that green capital is an apolitical and ultimately dissatisfying stand-in for the thing that we dare not take up because, as we know, it is just too hard. Instead, real climate change solutions—those that might significantly alter existing wealthy-world lifestyles—are substituted for the doable, low-hanging fruit.

A similar thing might therefore be said of Kuli Kuli—that it is a weak stand-in for addressing crushing, unrelenting poverty, all the more because it forwards healthy lifestyles for those who are complicit in it, if not directly responsible. Developing entrepreneurial capacities is a particularly apolitical approach to hunger, as Li (2007) might put it, rendering the problem of poverty not only technical but commodifiable and effectively "ignoring the circumstances through which one social group impoverishes another" (p. 7). For that matter, rendering snack food as medicine, in what McDonell (2015) calls a curative model, is depoliticizing in another way, extracting food from its social and cultural context as if moringa's sole meaning is set of curative nutrients—its superfoods status (also Scrinis 2013). Nevertheless, it is precisely these depoliticizing moves that make Kuli Kuli—and many other superfoods built on similar schemes—investable. Selling health in a bar promises a flow of capital while maintaining a promise of broader impact for those up the supply chain. This, then, is its own kind of solutionism—not a solutionism that precedes the problem, but a solutionism that diminishes the problem—and in setting up the potential for failure for those whose situation is most dire may ultimately do more harm than good.

Notes

1   According to the website, Kuli Kuli's mission is to improve nutrition and livelihoods worldwide. "Our vision is to work with women-led farming cooperatives all over the world to drive economic growth, women's empowerment, and sustainable agricultural development. We are creating a world where everyone has the resources and knowledge to access the nutritional power of moringa. By rejuvenating moringa as a tool for nutritional security, we hope a new generation will imagine a world without hunger" (Kuli Kuli 2019).

2   The same could be said of organics and fair trade, but at least those labels are underpinned by identifiable and verifiable processes that attest to specific social

and environmental outcomes, as flawed as these processes are. See Dolan 2010; Goodman 2004; and Guthman 2004.

3   That the company was talking about biodiversity and hiring practices in the same breath is noteworthy as well.

4   But unlike quinoa, moringa is not a staple of many people's diets. It was not widely grown and instead used primarily medicinally.

5   I have nothing against yoga or even yoga pants. This is just a shorthand for a particular demographic.

6

The Miracle Crop as Boundary Object: Quinoa's Rise as a "Neglected and Under-Utilized Species"

Emma McDonell

Over the past decade, quinoa has become famous as the archetypical consumer "superfood." A product mostly unknown beyond the Andes until recently, wealthy health-conscious eaters across the globe now prize the grain for its nutritional properties. Yet today's elite consumers were not the first to imagine quinoa's ability to work miracles. In the mid-twentieth century, international development experts began envisioning quinoa as a miracle crop with the potential to "cure" problems of underdevelopment. Quinoa's curative powers were imagined not as acting on the individual consumer body, but as working on the social body (see LeBlanc, this volume, for a related case). Quinoa offered both a nutritional miracle and a potential solution to broader economic and sociopolitical dilemmas. Within the international development community, quinoa became a potential answer to malnutrition in the Andes, a global hunger curative, a lucrative export that could alleviate Andean poverty, and a climate change adaptation crop for use in drought-prone environments across the world. A one-size-fits-all development miracle crop, quinoa seemed capable of solving any and all complex development dilemma. While numerous development actors have seen unrealized potential in quinoa, what exactly that potential is—what problems it ought to solve—varies widely.

Some visions of quinoa's potential are incompatible. For instance, if quinoa is to solve malnutrition in Andean countries, its price needs to be low enough that urban poor can afford it. If it is positioned to alleviate poverty among small farmers in the Andes as a high-value export crop, the price needs to be high. And if farmers in the highlands are to earn sufficient income from quinoa production, expanding production into new areas outside the Andes in the name of climate change adaptation will likely undermine this goal, foreclosing Andean farmers' competitive advantage in global markets.

New visions of quinoa's potential do not replace existing visions. They co-exist, at times awkwardly. Stories about quinoa's potential were not successive in a simple way—they've built upon each other. Because all parties agreed that quinoa has "unrealized potential," the incompatibilities between these narratives went (and continue to go) mostly undiscussed. The miracle crop is an incredibly effective boundary object, in part because of its basis in potential.

This chapter examines the multiple promissory narratives (cf. Brown and Michael 2003) circulating about quinoa's unrealized potential as a development tool. Like other development miracle crops, quinoa's unrealized potential serves as a boundary object (cf. Star 1985) that helps forge collaborations among diverse constituencies by allowing incompatible discourses to co-exist without open conflict. Agreement about quinoa's unrealized potential obscures the lack of consensus about quinoa's proper future: the politics of who ought to benefit from quinoa and how.

First, I trace how quinoa became legible to the international development community through the rise of concept of the neglected and under-utilized species. I then summarize the main visions of quinoa's potential, highlighting overlaps and inconsistencies between each story. I conclude by analyzing the United Nations' declaration of 2013 as the International Year of Quinoa (IYQ) as an instance when the boundary object quality of quinoa's development potential peaks and then starts to break down, commenting on the centrality and the danger of boundary objects in international development work.

From *comida de indios* to Under-Utilized Crop

Domesticated near the shores of Lake Titicaca some 5,000 years ago, quinoa has long been physically and symbolically mapped onto the Andean highlands.[1] Until recently, quinoa production and consumption took place almost exclusively in the Andes and the grain is intimately connected to regional identities and cultural practices.

Because of its connection to indigenous Andeans, quinoa came to be highly stigmatized over the course of Spanish colonialism. After an initial period of symbolic instability, Spanish colonists came to see quinoa as a *comida de indios* ("Indian food")—quinoa consumption became one of a number of food practices used to differentiate colonized and colonizers in the region, including consuming guinea pig, alpaca meat, and even barley, which was actually introduced from the Old World (Dietler 2006; Earle 2014; García 2010; Markowitz 2012; Weismantel 2000).[2]

In part because of this stigma, the mainstream scientific community ignored quinoa at first, paralleling early twentieth-century European attitudes toward maize consumption in Mexico. Maize consumption was inhibiting American "development"—a belief that explained why the wheat-consuming Europeans ruled the world (Pilcher 1998). The coloniality of power—the obvious superiority of all things European—made it bizarre to study the potential of a grain consumed almost exclusively by Indians (Quijano 1999). By definition, Indian foods were connected to the past, not the future.

Despite this, quinoa caught the attention of a small group of unconventional Andean nutrition scientists in the 1930s. A study conducted in Argentina in the 1930s found that bread made from a mix of wheat and quinoa flour was more nutritious than wheat bread (Viñas 1953), something confirmed by Bolivian chemists in the late 1940s who saw potential for quinoa as a military ration (Alcázar 1948). Studies conducted primarily in Peru in the late 1940s documented quinoa's amino acid profile, demonstrating the high quality of the protein in the grain when compared to dairy products (see White et al. 1955). This research focused on measuring quinoa's protein, a dynamic reflecting protein's status as that moment's charismatic nutrient (Kimura 2013) and a related global "protein gap" discourse (see LeBlanc, this volume).

Quinoa, they thought, might be a solution to malnutrition in the Andes, a problem increasingly identified in reports published by the emerging international development community:

> Increasing the production area and consumption [of quinoa] deserve to be considered by the [Peruvian] state as a nutritional policy, today more than ever, as it is a high-quality food, especially for the Andean population, whose nutritional deficiencies and particularly the ingestion of protein substances are always so notorious. The development of a joint plan to increase both quinoa cultivation and propaganda of quinoa's nutritional virtues will result in an increase in its use, with the benefits that can be expected from all this.
>
> (Viñas 1953, 180)

Meanwhile, other reports on malnutrition in the Andes found that populations were exceeding recommended protein consumption quotas and that vitamin A and calcium were the primary "deficiencies." Indeed, development experts are trained to frame problems around existing solutions (Ferguson 1990; Li 2007; see Guthman, this volume).

Scientific interest in quinoa gradually expanded in the 1950s and 1960s, a dynamic marked by the emergence of collaborations between Peruvian scientists and researchers at Harvard University and University of Iowa along with funding from the United States Department of Agriculture (USDA) and the US National Research Council for their work (Alvistur et al. 1953). A handful of quinoa-related research projects were conducted in the United States: the USDA funded (unsuccessful) experimental plots in Colorado (Eiselen 1956), experimental plots were cultivated in Europe (Cutler 1954), and a doctoral dissertation on quinoa's origins and taxonomy was published in 1968 (Nelson 1968). Word of a mysterious and intriguing nutritional wonder grain made sporadic appearances in US media.

While awareness in quinoa's potential grew among nutrition scientists and agronomists, the international development community was slower to incorporate quinoa into actual "development projects." Agricultural development and global hunger discourses at the time centered on commodity crops and neo-Malthusian ideas about productivity and food shortage, making quinoa's role unclear. There was no existing category quinoa fit into. Indeed, native crops without strong markets were precisely the species the development apparatus was looking to replace.

This changed in the 1970s when a group of vangaurdist development experts frustrated with the Green Revolution zeitgeist created the idea of the "under-exploited crop." Variously referred to as minor crops, crops with potential, orphan crops, promising crops, or under-exploited crops, and as the discourse consolidated, "neglected and under-utilized species" (commonly with the acronym "NUS"), the category included species (crops and domesticated animals) that had received little attention in the global development community but had "potential." An ad hoc panel of US-based researchers, including botanists, pharmaceutical researchers, and biochemists, published an influential volume on NUS with the National Academy of Sciences (NAS) in 1975, titled *Underexploited Tropical Plants with Promising Economic Value.* The opening line describes their vision:

> This is a report on plants that show promise for improving the quality of life in tropical areas. Because the countries in this zone contain most of the world's low-income populations this report is addressed to those government

administrators, technical assistance personal [*Sic*], and researchers in agriculture, nutrition, and related disciplines who are concerned with helping developing countries achieve a more efficient and balanced exploitation of their biological resources.

(1975, v)

The book features a diverse array of species including quinoa, amaranth, spirulina, teff, winged beans, and acacia (many of which are today marketed as consumer superfoods), with their described "potential" ranging widely. *Acacia albida*, for instance, is imagined as a potential cure for soil infertility and as improved forage in Africa while authors envision the burutí palm as a source of oil and starch for food, wine, timber, cork, and industrial fiber for twine, sacking nets, and hammocks (133).

The development experts who disseminated this discourse criticized how a small number of species dominated agricultural development, framing this issue within a neo-Malthusian crisis narrative:

> The strain on world resources posed by rapid population growth, dwindling supplies of nonrenewable resources, and shortages of food puts economic botany in the mainstream of human concerns. Throughout human history man has used some 3,000 plant species for food ... But over the centuries the tendency has been to concentrate on fewer and fewer. Today, most of the people in the world are fed by about 20 crops ... These plants are the main bulwark between mankind and starvation.

(1975, 1)

The Green Revolution's emphasis on a small number of crops was misguided, they argued, and begged a catastrophe of epic proportions.

The "alternative-ness" of the vision is in the way that these "experts" saw potential in very same crops the Green Revolution model sought to supplant. The NAS's 1975 book even explains the neglect of these crops as an issue of the coloniality of power (Quijano 1999) as it manifests in research priorities:

> The apparent advantages of staple plants over minor tropical plants often result only from the disproportionate research attention they have been given. Many indigenous species may possess equal merit, but were disregarded during the colonial era when consumer demands in European countries largely determined the cultivation (and research) priorities in tropical agriculture. The crops selected ... received considerable research and extension. Even after independence, the pattern of concentrating on a few crops changed little.

Furthermore, as indigenous scientists were generally trained in the institutions
of temperate-zone countries they had little interest in studying tropical species.

(NAS 1975, 1)

The NUS concept was based on a critique of the way colonialism shapes
knowledge production and the resulting agricultural science priorities. By
heralding crops devalued by colonialist agricultural politics and the consequent
development apparatus as key development tools, proponents of the discourse
invert the linking non-European ways of being with the past while implicitly
questioning the legitimacy of the very systems that led to the devaluation
("disappearance") of these crops. Of course, this critique is limited to the issue
of a perceived lack of attention paid to crops like quinoa. The NUS discourse
reproduces other colonialist logics, and it's worth noting that this critique never
became dominant.

The idea was that more research—more bioprospecting (my term not
theirs)—was needed to find crop species equipped to solve the twin issues of
increasingly vulnerable monocultural agricultural systems and food shortages
that the authors see as defining dilemmas of the moment: "Man has only
just begun to take stock of the chemical and genetic possibilities in the plant
kingdom. Now we must scrutinize the thousands of plant species, many of
which are still untested and some as yet unidentified" (1975, 1). The report
went on to talk about these crops as in peril of extinction, and to propose
the development of new infrastructure: "Careful preservation and thorough
cataloguing are particularly important for little-known plants such as those
described in the report ... Potential breeding stocks, clones, and cultivars will
otherwise become extinct" (1975, 3). The NUS fantasy of finding a species that
can solve development problems overlaps with the bioprospecting discourse
that emerged in the 1990s, which also relied on the construction of potential
and extinction panics (Greene 2004; Hayden 2003). In other words, we might
find the "curative" (McDonell 2015) or antidote to development ills that high-
yield varieties had not provided, but only if we acted fast.[3] Indeed, generating
this fear of loss and endangerment served to activate the potentiality, creating
a sense of urgency around protecting these crops.

During the 1980s, the discourse spread into US-based development
institutions and research networks in what was then labeled the "developing
world." Some university researchers began to think about their research through
this framework, as we see in a 1987 report from the University of Minnesota
Agricultural Experiment Station titled "Amaranth, Quinoa, Ragi, Tef, and

Niger: Tiny Seeds of Ancient History and Modern Interest"—a convergence of crops that only makes sense if one sees them as having in common a quality of underutilization (Robinson 1986). In 1986, the United Nations' Food and Agriculture Organization (FAO) organized a meeting about "Underexploited Andean Crops of Nutritional Value" in Santiago, Chile, and by 1988 the International Centre for Underutilized Crops was established in London, a center dedicated to the study of NUS. That same year, Purdue University hosted a first symposium on new crops.[4] In 1990, an acclaimed Peruvian agronomist partnered with researchers at the FAO to publish *Underexploited Andean Crops and Their Contribution to Nutrition*, a book discussing the potential of quinoa and a handful of other Andean crops and what needed to be done to properly utilize them.

But what exactly was the promise of these crops? What "utility" was not being utilized? What would it look like to properly utilize their potential? The early NUS texts are unclear and, at times, contradictory. In the 1975 NAS book, quinoa is at once pitched as under-utilized for income generation in developing countries (i.e., a potential export crop), malnutrition alleviation in the Andes, and global malnutrition relief. In other words, the problems that these species could solve were numerous. The authors clearly did not agree on what they should be used for, only that they were not sufficiently utilized.

It makes sense that quinoa's classification as an under-utilized crop came about when experts outside the Andes "discovered" quinoa.[5] The claim that quinoa was under-utilized would strike anyone familiar with the Andes as a puzzling proposition given that millions of people eat it on a daily basis, and those who consume it are primarily the poor people that the volume authors claim to want to assist. Stigmatized, yes. But under-utilized, no. Indeed, the authors at one point seem to assert that quinoa has disappeared: "The Spanish introduced wheat and barley and focused agriculture research only on those crops, which eventually displaced quinoa" (1975, 2). At a later point in the book they present information that demonstrates that it has not "disappeared," but still engage in a discourse of disappearance throughout the text.

Quinoa's framing as a neglected and under-utilized crop—the vagueness of its proclaimed development *potential*—allowed stories about its potential development applications to multiply. Hype around quinoa's potential in turn brought together expert communities who usually operated in separate institutional realms: nutrition scientists, agronomists, entrepreneurs, biodiversity experts, rural development experts, Latin America-oriented development organizations like the Inter-American Development Bank and globally oriented ones like Biodiversity International. Four primary visions of quinoa's development potential have since emerged: quinoa as a malnutrition palliative in the Andes, quinoa as a global hunger curative, quinoa as a poverty alleviation tool in the Andes, and quinoa as a global climate change adaptation crop.

Visions of Potential

Quinoa as a Malnutrition Palliative in the Andes

When scientists and development experts based in Andean countries initially began studying quinoa in the 1940s and 1950s, they imagined quinoa as a solution to malnutrition in the Andes. In 1949, *The New York Times* published an article about the mysterious miracle grain, titled "Latin Nations See New Food in Quinoa: U.N. Group to Study Nutritive Value of Ancient Inca Plant for Upland Indigenes." The article discusses how Bolivia, at the conference on nutrition in Latin America, made a formal request to the United Nations' FAO to study quinoa, "an ancient plant considered as sacred by the Incas, as a possible supplementary food in the Hemisphere to combat malnutrition" (Bracker 1948). Thus, quinoa's development potential first came to be known among actors in the international development world through calls for its application to malnutrition in Latin America.

While reports about malnutrition in the Andes did not single out protein as a problem, quinoa's protein content was frequently touted as its key to alleviating malnutrition in the region. Both Andean researchers and development experts shared this vision. Edward Weber, the senior program officer for the Agriculture, Food and Nutrition Sciences Division of the Latin American International Development Research Centre's regional office in Bogotá penned an article in *Nature* framing quinoa as an answer to the "acute protein shortage" in the Andes: "Researchers in a number of Latin American countries are looking at a crop first cultivated by the ancient Incas and then neglected for centuries, as a possible answer to the Andean region's acute shortage of locally produced food protein" (Weber 1978, 486). Of course, this claim of neglect in Latin American countries is quite strange given its prominence in local diets.

For some, the nutritional deficiencies were directly connected with the "modernization" of diets that had led to the replacement of foods like quinoa with less nutritious staples (Ferroni 1982). For others, this was directly connected to the rise of cheap imported wheat from the United States (Arévalo and Maisch 1986; Cusack 1984; Tapia 2000). No matter what caused the problem, quinoa advocates agreed that quinoa was the solution. The influence of dependency theory and import substitution industrialization in Latin America made using a local crop an attractive and politically salient way to solve nutritional problems than continued reliance on cheap wheat imports from the United States.

Peru's nutritional assistance program was one of the first major purchasers of commercial quinoa in the 1990s. And while much has been made of the program's lofty discourse around emphasizing local ingredients and its failure to do so, Peru's national school breakfast program, Qali Warma, does continue to purchase some quinoa.

It's common in public discourse in Andean countries to hear laments that people do not eat as much quinoa as "they should." It is indeed an irony that in a country apparently abounding in nutritional miracle foods there is a high incidence of malnutrition. The notion that quinoa is not living up to its potential to eliminate malnutrition in the Andes is pervasive among development experts and among the general public in Peru. Mario Tapia explains this contradiction in a 2000 chapter on NUS in Latin America:

> Latin America, despite many efforts, has around 64 million chronically malnourished persons, representing 13% of the population. This situation contrasts with the potentiality of its agriculture and the grand variety of genetic resources, among them, Andean crops. Some of these, like potatoes and corn, have reached global diffusion and constitute a basic staple in many countries. However, other crops remain underexploited, representing a major opportunity to increase the nutritional base.
>
> (Tapia 2000)

These reports, in typical solutionist fashion, have little to say about the complex drivers of malnutrition and instead point to increased research on and dissemination of under-utilized crops as solutions. It's worth noting that social scientists have shown again and again that the cause of malnutrition is not the failure of agriculture but issues of power and structural inequality (Sen 1981). These miracle food stories are incredibly effective in depoliticizing malnutrition (McDonell 2015).

Proponents of this vision point to outdated production methods and low productivity as the cause of the insufficient quinoa supply, which they consider the chief obstacle to utilizing quinoa to solve malnutrition in the Andes.

Increasing quinoa production in the name of solving malnutrition in the Andes was taken up by governments, at least discursively, starting in the 1930s when the earliest studies about quinoa were published. In 1937, *The New York Times* published a special cable from Lima, titled "Peru Backs Cultivation of Quinoa as a Cereal," which briefed readers on an effort by the Peruvian government to increase production of quinoa and highlighted a study comparing Argentine wheat to quinoa-based bread as the government's motive for this move (*The New York Times* 1937). Any agricultural economist would have been able to tell them that increasing production would further reduce the already low farm-gate price, something that would contradict the goal of turning quinoa production into an income-generating activity for highland farmers. And based on the low price quinoa maintained during the twentieth century, the problem was not insufficient supply but insufficient demand.

In the 1970s, during the leftist government of Juan Velasco Alvarado whose *dependencista* vision demonized US wheat imports, the Peruvian government began paying more attention to quinoa. A 1973 Ministry of Agriculture report, titled "Economic Aspects of Quinoa Cultivation," evaluates the costs of quinoa production in the Puno region, introducing the importance of the study with regard to nutrition: "Moreover, [quinoa] is a product rich in vitamins and proteins, necessary for human nutrition" (Ministerio de Agricultura 1973, iii). In neighboring Bolivia, the leftist military government of Hugo Banzer passed a law obligating bread flours to contain a minimum of 5 percent quinoa flour in 1974, though the law has never been enforced.

The vision of quinoa as a cure for malnutrition in the Andes continues today. While few quinoa-related development projects explicitly focus on promoting its consumption for malnutrition alleviation (in the Andes, projects focus much more on export markets today), they generally justify their work in relation to the narrative of the role quinoa consumption could play in eradicating hunger in the Andes. For instance, the McKnight Foundation's crop research partnership with the Bolivian development research group, PROINPA, frames the importance of their project around hunger in the Andes: "The people of the high Andes of Bolivia and Peru have the lowest per-capita income in South America. They suffer from economic isolation and widespread malnutrition," opens their project description (McKnight Foundation 2020). More recently, quinoa has been framed as the solution to the rising rates of anemia in the Andean highlands as well (Andina n.d.). Even as efforts to apply quinoa to solving malnutrition in the Andes wane, the discourse itself remains strong.

Quinoa as Global Malnutrition Curative

As fears about a global food crisis intensified in the 1970s and development actors outside the Andes grew more familiar with quinoa, more development actors came to see quinoa as a solution to malnutrition at a global level. In the justifications for the second Chenopod Convention in Potosí, Bolivia, in 1976, Andean researchers reference multiple visions of quinoa's potential:

> Considering that the cultivation of Chenopodiaceae constitutes a central part of agricultural production for large sectors of the Andean campesino population; That quinoa and kañiwa are two species that have fundamental importance in the lives of Andean peoples, constituting basic elements of their alimentation; *That the global crisis in food production, particularly with respect to cereals and the demographic explosion, constitutes imminent danger for the wellbeing of humanity and thus requires finding new food supplies;* That it is of upmost importance to solve the problems of quinoa commercialization, consumption, and industrialization with the goal of ensuring a secure and profitable market; That the adoption of policies that strengthen production of these species is in the national interest in general and interest of the producers of Chenopodioideae in particular.
>
> (1976, 8; emphasis added)

While the NAS's first volume had proposed many possible futures for what properly "utilizing" quinoa would look like, by the publication of NAS's 1989 book on Andean NUS, *Lost Crop of the Incas: Little-Known Plants of the Andes with Promise for Worldwide Cultivation*, the goal was global expansion. Indeed, an ode to quinoa opening the 1978 Chenopod Convention proceedings shows that the idea that quinoa had a global role was already common: "Quinoa, a noble plant that was a food for our esteemed Aymara and Quechua cultures, is called to complete an important role in the solution of the world's nutritional problems" (1976, 7).

Yet, the authors appear to struggle with allegiances. As they explain in the preface:

> This report has been written for dissemination to administrators, entrepreneurs, and researchers in developing countries as well as in North America, Europe, and Australasia … The ultimate aim is to raise nutritional levels and create economic opportunities, particularly in the Andes. The report, however, deliberately describes the promise of these plants for markets in industrialized nations. It is

in these countries (where a concentration of research facilities and discretionary research funds may be found) that many important research contributions are likely to be made.

(1989, vi)

They at once see NUS like quinoa as having "promise for worldwide cultivation" while asserting that their ultimate aim is to encourage "development" in the Andean countries, where these plants originate.

The work of expanding quinoa production into new areas had actually begun much earlier, when seeds obtained from the Kew Royal Botanical Gardens in Britain were introduced to Kenya in 1935 (Elmer 1942). Trials took place in a number of countries during the twentieth century and became more systematic in the 1990s. Starting in 1996, researchers from Peru, Denmark, and the FAO collaborated to conduct the "American and European Test of Quinoa" and a similar program by International Potato Center (CIP) and the Danish development cooperation was also carried out in the 1990s. The stated goal of this effort was directly related to malnutrition:

[The aim is] to improve the production conditions and nutrition of the general population, above all in areas with climactic challenges, as quinoa has major advantages and possibilities both for the nourishment of humans and animal ... and because of its ability to adapt to new areas and the ease with which the crop can be produced with modern and mechanized production.

(Mujica et al. 2001b)

Quinoa was imagined as a global malnutrition curative not only because of its nutritional content but also because of the supposed ease with which it could be adapted to diverse environments.[6]

This vision of quinoa as a global hunger curative (cf. McDonell 2015) has recently grown in popularity. In 2011, the FAO published *Quinoa, an Ancient Crop to Contribute to World Food Security*, a report that foreshadows the declaration of 2013 as the United Nations' IYQ. The opening lines of the report make clear the vision:

[The report] is an updated and detailed compilation of the nutritional benefits and agricultural versatility of quinoa; the expansion of the crop to other continents and showing that it is a crop with high potential to contribute to food security in various Regions worldwide, especially in those countries where the population does not have access to protein sources or where production conditions are limited by low humidity, reduced availability of inputs, and aridity.

(PROINPA/FAO 2011)

Here, the genetic diversity within the species is the crucial quality that allows for the framing of quinoa expansion potential. The genetic "material" exists for developing new quinoa varieties adapted to specific environments (Bazile 2014).

Yet, the visions overlap in confusing ways. The National Research Council's *Lost Crops of the Incas* explicitly advocates "worldwide cultivation" and discusses at length the potential of cultivating these plants in the United States and Europe. Yet the authors at one point claim that their ultimate goal is to help relieve nutritional problems in the Andes. The claim that introducing these crops to the United States and Europe offers the technical expertise and facilities to realize quinoa's potential for the Andes is dubious given the patterns of how plant resources are extracted from the Global South and often "improved" in the Global North, patented, and sold back to the South (Kloppenburg 1988). Yet this shifty logic is never discussed or debated. Instead, the agreement about quinoa's unrealized potential allows for inconsistencies like this to fade into the background.

Quinoa as Poverty Alleviation in the Andean Highlands

Food experts said that, [*sic*] just as the history of such basic foods as potatoes, tomatoes and possibly corn, could be traced back to South America, it was conceivable that some day quinoa, through modern cultivation, might occupy a major role in feeding the Upland Indians, whose needs are among the greatest in the Americas, Bolivian delegates tended to regard the plant as an eventual export commodity. Others felt that this opinion was premature, but, agreed that the plant merited the fullest development in terms of the local populations' needs.

(Bracker 1948)

Even at the FAO's first summit about malnutrition in Latin America, some experts in the nascent international development community had set their sights on quinoa as an export commodity. Yet this vision would not gain prominence until the late 1970s, when rural incomes (and lack thereof) came to the fore of the international development agenda (Macekura 2015, 91–136).

Quinoa was envisioned a potential cash crop—an "income-generating activity" for farmers in the Andean highlands. In addition to the shift from thinking about jobs to income-generating activities in development globally, two other developments contribute to the emergence of this new problem/solution story: the questions arising from the agrarian reform in Peru and the emergence of demand for quinoa in the United States in the 1980s.

Peru's top-down agrarian reform was implemented over the course of the 1970s by the leftist military government of Juan Velasco Alvarado and, after the fall of his administration, that of Francisco Morales Bermúdez. This "revolution from above" expropriated thousands of hectares of land from the semi-feudalist hacienda system, converting much of this land into complex institutional arrangements, including producer cooperatives and peasant communities (Mayer 2009). The question of how these newly independent farmers and cooperative businesses would sustain themselves was pressing, and many development actors portrayed the "stunted" capitalization of the altiplano as a key obstacle to their success. In Peru, the dream of profitable quinoa production arose in part in relation to the reorganization of land tenure arrangements and the sociopolitical order in the highlands.

One of the first development projects to look into quinoa as a cash crop took place between 1977 and 1978 in Puno, Peru. The project, called "Fostering the Agroindustrial Production of Quinoa in Puno," was funded by the Inter-American Institute for Cooperation on Agriculture (IICA), and involved Peru's Ministry of Agriculture and Alimentation and UNICEF, among others (Egoávil et al. 1979). The framing of the project makes clear that the authors see their effort to improve the commercial production of quinoa as a service to farmers (as income generation) *and* as a malnutrition alleviation strategy in Peru:

> One of the basic problems of the food sector is low food production and dependence on foreign sources for basic food products and raw material. There is also a serious caloric disorder or lack of balance in nutritional levels, which is accentuated in the Puno sector of the country ... Quinoa has been considered a product which could help accomplish these objectives at regional and national levels, since there are 12,000 hectares of this crop already being cultivated and there is an estimated potential for 45,000 additional hectares.

> (Egoávil et al. 1979, 115)

The project marked the first effort to delineate the obstacles to a lucrative commercial quinoa industry in Peru. The project was influential in the national agricultural development community, inspiring a conversation around "improving" quinoa production and marketability. Studies looked into technologies to overcome the obstacles identified in the project, such as machinery for removing the bitter saponin coating from quinoa grains (Torres 1980). Others focused on developing networks to sell "improved" quinoa seeds.

While the reports focus on the "production obstacles," various development agents who were working at this time told me that the fundamental issue was a lack of demand. This was clear when I spoke with Gustavo, one of the pioneers of commercial quinoa production in Puno. He started an NGO in the early 1990s that organized farmers into producer associations (which make buying quinoa more efficient) and trained them in "improved methods" while offering credit for access to tractors and classes in "comportment" and "hygiene." He told me that the reason farmers were not planting much quinoa was that there was no demand. The pioneers of this vision of quinoa alleviating poverty in the altiplano were working from quinoa's *potential* as a profitable crop, not the reality at the time in which quinoa was cheap and undesirable.

> G: The peasants [campesinos] cultivated very little quinoa. Very very little
>   quinoa ...
> E: Only for eating in the home?
> G: It was for the most part for auto-consumption, subsistence.
> E: They only grew potatoes at the time for income then?
> G: Yes, they cultivated way more potato, also mostly just to eat themselves,
>   and they cultivated lots of kinds of potatoes. They had a ton of biodiversity.
>   In general, they cultivated crops to eat themselves and sold very little of
>   their harvest. And at the time the arroba cost between eight and ten soles.[7]
>   Quinoa was super cheap. And besides this, there was no "quinoa boom." No
>   one knew about quinoa. Not in Lima, not in Europe, not in the US, nothing
>   like that. And when we did a study about quinoa among different social
>   strata in Lima, Arequipa, Cusco, and Trujillo, people said that quinoa was
>   for Indians. People saw it as chicken scratch.

When some US consumers began taking an interest in quinoa in the early 1980s, some development actors took notice. A small export market developed, primarily with Bolivian quinoa. Quinoa began trickling into health food markets across the United States after a small import venture based out of Boulder, Colorado, which would become Ancient Harvest, began selling quinoa in 1 lb bags.[8] By the mid-1980s, the grain had a dedicated group of consumers among New Age dieters.[9] While quinoa did not at the time attract quite the attention of spirulina—the alternative health food superfood darling of the time—a number of laudatory introductions to the "lost crop of the Incas" began circulating in health media outlets and lefty environmentalist publications like *The Ecologist*. The Natural Food Institute wrote about quinoa in its pamphlet "Wonder Crops" in 1985. In 1988, Rebecca Wood, author of *The Whole Foods Encyclopedia*, published *Quinoa: The Supergrain* with a cover selling quinoa as "the sacred wonder grain of the ancient Incas," beckoning readers with an offer to "discover the ancient grain that gives you new energy and revitalizes your favorite recipes." In 1988, *The New York Times* published a couple of basic quinoa recipes and its dining section featured an article on a Thanksgiving cookout that featured a quinoa dish—signs that quinoa's transition from obscure hippie food to upscale "yuppie food" (cf. Guthman 2003) was apace.

Growing interest among foreign consumers caught the attention of some development experts concerned with the lack of income opportunities for rural families in the altiplano. After a decade of civil war that had devastated rural communities in the highlands in particular, development actors attuned to the region perceived an urgent need for programs that could revive rural economies. In the early 1990s, a handful of organizations working on agricultural development in the altiplano began to imagine quinoa as potentially lucrative cash crop that could provide income to impoverished farmers who for the most part did not have markets for their crops.

The chief obstacles from the perspective of the development actors who shared this vision were what they defined as the "low quality production" and disorganized farmers. Farmers used techniques that made sense in a complex biodiverse agricultural system in the context of the harsh Andean climate but were not using "modern" methods such as plows, furrows, chemical fertilizers, or improved seeds. Farmers did not have access to technology such as tractors or mechanizing threshers that would make increased productivity possible and produce a more homogenous product. Moreover, farmers were cultivating many kinds of quinoa, a practice inimical to commodification.

In the early 1990s, two NGOs began working with farmers in different parts of Puno to organize farmers into producer associations and offer technical assistance and credit. The idea was that if they organized the farmers into produce association, they could more easily train them while also pooling product to facilitate formal quinoa markets. It was not easy to convince farmers to implement "modern" farming methods when the price was so low. Planting quinoa in furrows, using improved seeds, and renting tractors required much more time, effort, skills, and economic investment, and not all farmers were convinced this would work out well.

But the idea that focusing on quinoa export would undermine the goal of making it more available for solving nutrition problems in the Andes was not common initially. One of the early pioneers of quinoa export, a founder of the Quinoa Corporation, imagines quinoa as both an export crop *and* a malnutrition miracle both in the Andes and globally in a 1984 article in *The Ecologist*. He concludes by arguing that developing export markets might actually be the best way to solve malnutrition in the Andes.

> Although lack of a cultivation tradition and complete unfamiliarity with quinua
> [*sic*] are greater problems in countries outside of the Andes, other countries

do not face historical and cultural prejudices against quinua [*sic*]. If successful transplants can be made, quinua [*sic*] products may be readily accepted, moreover a developed country health food market is a logical place to introduce a new food crop like quinua [*sic*], especially in view of its excellent nutritional quality. This considerable market ($2.4 billion in the United States) is made up of a clientele which values nutrition, is receptive to new products, and is intrigued by the unfamiliar and exotic. This market has been the starting point for the entry of many new products into the mainstream US market. Opening a US market could be a positive stimulus for improving the South American market for quinua [*sic*], which is the weakest link in the South American system. It can lead to increased consumer product variety and attractiveness, which in turn can have a significant demonstration impact on the urban populations of Andean countries. A Peruvian researcher once remarked that the shortest marketing route for quinua [*sic*] from Cuzco (the former capital of the Inca Empire) to Lima (the modern capital of Peru) may be through the US health food market. In a modern world interlocked by instant communications and mass media, increased consumer demand may be more easily transferred than sophisticated production and processing technology.

(Cusack 1984, 31)

For Cusack, there is no tension between developing quinoa export markets and the use of quinoa to alleviate malnutrition in the Andes. Instead, he sees developing export production as ultimately serving the end of improving nutritional deficiencies in Andean countries, a rather odd logic, but one that is quite common in the discourse around quinoa's many potentials.

When export demand picked up in the early 2000s, increased effort went into developing export production in Puno and eventually in other regions of Peru. Much of this work was framed as poverty alleviation in the Andes, despite the fact that this was a money-making venture for lots of actors, including middlemen, development agents, exporters, marketing agencies, and all of the other actors that benefit from a commodity boom. But the story that quinoa could solve and was solving poverty in the high Andes became increasingly popular as quinoa demand outside the Andes began to spike around 2008.

Quinoa as a Climate Change Adaptation Tool

Conversations about climate change gained urgency in the agricultural development world over the course of the early 2000s, anticipating increasing climate uncertainty and more frequent climate extremes. The World Bank and the FAO published numerous reports about this issue at the global scale, while locally oriented NGOs and development organizations began looking into the specific ways climate change could manifest in different regions, and what "adapting" might entail.

The dilemma was at once about maintaining food supply in affected regions and about buffering the shocks of extreme weather events and changing climate patterns for people practicing "land-based livelihoods," like farming and fishing. As a language of adaptation came to dominate these discussions at the global level (Orlove 2009), the search for climate adaptation tools intensified.

Climate change adaptation was added to the list of quinoa's imagined "utilities." While quinoa's hardiness had been celebrated previously, here, quinoa's ability to withstand environmental extremes (soils, rainfall, temperature, and altitude) and tolerance to frost, drought, and salinity took on new meaning (Mujica et al. 2001a; Ruiz et al. 2014; Vega-Gálvez et al. 2010). Research about quinoa's adaptability and hardiness became the basis for building quinoa's potentiality as a climate change adaptation mechanism.

In 2011, Biodiversity International organized a conference called "On-farm Conservation of Neglected and Underutilized Species: Status, Trends and Novel Approaches to Cope with Climate Change" (Padulosi et al. 2011). Quinoa was the conference star, and immediately thereafter multiple research groups began using quinoa as a climate change adaptation crop in sub-Saharan Africa. Then, a prominent journal article published in 2013 reviewed existing research and the prospect for quinoa as a climate change adaptation crop outside the Andes, using research on quinoa's tolerance for salinic soils along with its ability to withstand drought and extreme cold to build this potential (Ruiz et al. 2014).

This idea gained more momentum with the 2016 conference in Dubai called "Quinoa for Future Food and Nutrition Security in Marginal Environments," attended mostly by Middle Eastern researchers and a handful of South American researchers who had bought into this vision. The stated goal of the event was "to provide a unique platform for discussions on ecological, economic and social aspects related to introducing quinoa for sustainable agricultural production in marginal environments," a vague aim that allowed for diverse expert communities with different allegiances to co-exist.

This story is wholly disconnected from the global malnutrition problem-solution narrative. Indeed, part of quinoa's allure in climate change adaptation is its nutritional density *paired with* hardiness and adaptability. Yet, given the nature of the attendees and their presentation titles, which included the FAO Regional Representative for the Near East and North Africa and Director of the

Arab Bank for Economic Development in Africa as well as prominent agro-industrial business leaders and agronomists, it appears that there was a mix of people interested in adapting quinoa to "marginal environments" in the Middle East for commercial purposes and participants more interested in food security. The researchers I spoke with who had been in attendance remarked that there was no open debate about this issue.

It was sometimes surprising who got behind this vision of quinoa as a climate change adaptation tool. One well-known agronomist from Puno had been invited and offered an all-expenses-paid trip to Dubai to attend and present a paper. Despite the scorn he received from some local colleagues who saw expansion of quinoa production into new areas as undermining Andean quinoa export markets, he told me that he decided to attend the conference and offer his expertise on quinoa. He explained his reasoning to me as we chatted at a cafe shortly after he arrived home from Dubai:

> I'm very much against the backward idea that we have to keep quinoa for ourselves. But at the same time all these countries are using germplasm directly from Andean farmers and there needs to be some sort of mechanism to compensate them. We need to find a middle ground. There were very few Andeans at this conference—me and a guy from Bolivia and someone from Universidad la Molina in Lima—and I was the only person who brought up the compensation question. No one had even thought about it.

This rare moment of tension reveals the norm of tacit agreement across the different actors involved in "quinoa development." Because everyone agreed quinoa had unrealized potential, actors with divergent visions of what properly utilizing quinoa would look like could collaborate in spaces like the Dubai conference or on the transnational development projects that were working to realize all of these visions at the same time.

Clashing Visions: 2013, International Year of Quinoa

When the United Nations declared 2013 the IYQ, all of these visions combined into a single, highly contradictory agenda. The IYQ was a year-long series of events across the world, loosely organized by the FAO, all of which fell under the strategically vague aim of "promoting quinoa." This included culinary events showcasing inventive dishes using quinoa, events promoting quinoa as a high-value crop in areas where quinoa was not grown at the time, biodiversity competitions in the Andes highlands,[10] and some gala events involving politicians and high-level UN officials. The IYQ's stated goals included:

> Increasing the visibility of the great potential of quinoa to contribute to global food security, especially in countries where the population has no access to other protein sources or where production conditions are limiting ... Recognizing and valuing the contribution of the indigenous peoples of the Andes as custodians of quinoa who conserve this food for present and future generations ... [and] improving international cooperation and partnerships between public, private and nongovernmental organizations related to the cultivation of quinoa.
>
> (FAO 2013)

Based on the events included in the IYQ, the main goal appears to have been expanding quinoa production and consumption beyond the Andes. There were events all over the world, but in Peru most took place in Lima and only four official IYQ events took place in the highlands, where production is based. Yet quinoa industry actors in the highlands at the time saw any publicity as good publicity. After centuries of quinoa's denigration and devaluation, having important and powerful individuals and institutions recognize its value seemed good enough.

The Peruvian state seemed to align with the IYQ discourse and did not see promoting expansion of quinoa into other areas as a problem for smallholders:

> Quinoa, golden grain of the Andes, has become an extraordinary protagonist thanks for the contribution and support of diverse state entities as well as international organizations, that have seen in our Andean grain a potential for all of humanity. Thus, we are not just talking about the importance that quinoa has for Peru and the Peruvian peoples but for the rest of the countries.
>
> (MINAGRI 2014)

It's implied that highland farmers should "be proud" and thrilled with the recognition of their "conservation" work. The "indigenous peoples of the Andes" are considered stewards of quinoa, worthy of recognition for their work but nothing else.

The agreement about quinoa's unrealized potential, and the importance of realizing quinoa's potential, understood broadly, allowed actors with different interests and visions for quinoa's future to collaborate on planning and carrying out IYQ events. Those with drastically dissimilar agendas of quinoa's potential could agree on the importance of the IYQ, and the attention it brought to quinoa. No official IYQ event reports or videos demonstrated debate about the contradictions between the different projections of quinoa's utility. They share a eulogistic tone toward quinoa and its potential to contribute to so many causes. In fact, quinoa's potentials are commonly documented in list form in IYQ documents, demonstrating the fetishization of the solution—quinoa—before careful analysis of how exactly it would solve the various problems it is listed as a solution for (see Guthman, this volume).

Yet during and after the IYQ, some latent tensions did begin to surface, something that happens to all boundary objects (Star 1985, 2010). While official IYQ documents prioritize a vision of quinoa as a globally produced commodity that will help alleviate hunger at that scale, the heterogenous events that comprised the IYQ program show a latent struggle to define the future of quinoa. Proponents of each vision saw the IYQ as an opportunity to push forward their own agenda, and it became clear to some that the collaborations inspired by agreement about quinoa's potential were on shaky footing. The boundary object quality of quinoa's unrealized potential was challenged as discrepancies between visions were revealed through both the work of the IYQ and the sudden price fluctuations. Industry actors in Puno, including farmers, voiced discontent and anger about the expansion of quinoa production beyond the Andes, and many directly blamed the IYQ for promoting this. At the same time, the price spike was a boon for farmers in the Andes *and* a problem for poor Peruvian quinoa consumers (McDonell 2016). The incompatibility of quinoa's potential to solve malnutrition in the Andes and to alleviate poverty was becoming evident to some.

After the IYQ was over, actors involved in Puno's quinoa industry and more broadly Peru's quinoa industry almost unanimously agreed that the IYQ had been a sham, though the specific issues emphasized varied. For some, it was an attempt for national politicians like Nadine Heredia to take advantage of the quinoa boom for political interests and in doing to take advantage of quinoa farmers. For others, the problem was that the event did not prioritize the Andes and instead was framed around expanding production elsewhere, undercutting the industry. Indeed, the quinoa boom and bust revealed some of the problems previously left undiscussed: the problematic relationship between export price and consumption in producer countries, for instance.

Boundary objects are not only unstable, but they follow patterned trajectories. Over time, groups attempt to control them and, in doing so, provoke real disagreement. As dissonance increases, new categories and new boundary objects proliferate (Star 2010). The IYQ marked a shift in which quinoa's unrealized potential no longer worked as seamlessly as a boundary object. The contradictions between the disparate visions of quinoa's future become increasingly visible.

Conclusion: Miracle Crops as Boundary Objects

Like consumer superfoods, development miracle crops need "really good stories behind them," something the NUS discourse provides (see Guthman, this volume). In 2019, the FAO reaffirmed its commitment to utilizing under-utilized crops in an article titled "Once Neglected, These Traditional Crops Are Our New Rising Stars: How Overlooked and Underutilized Crops Are Getting Their Turn in the Spotlight." The article frames their potential around solving hunger, climate change adaptation, and export: "Traditional foods have been around for centuries, but have become neglected as more productive, profitable or improved crops replaced them in farming systems. Yet, many are highly nutritious, naturally climate resilient and even potentially valuable in global trade, making them a great ally for a Zero Hunger future" (2018). The story of the under-utilized miracle crop is a powerful story and a powerful boundary object. Even as the crop filling the slot will change (for example, of other crops that have filled this slot, see LeBlanc, this volume; McDonell 2015; Rao and Huggins 2017), the miracle crop slot will persist.

Tracing the competing visions of quinoa's future leaves us with the question of whose interests framing a crop as under-utilized—invoking miracle crop potential—serves. In the case of quinoa, the agreement around quinoa's development potential avoided debate of inconsistencies and contraditions. Boundary objects abound in development work because they justify reproducing and expanding the (quinoa) development apparatus. They encourage new projects, thereby offering new jobs for the development practitioners with previous experience (with quinoa), and facilitate the involvement of private sector actors without questioning their motives.

While the boundary object concept was developed to understand how scientists with different expertise collaborate and work to develop knowledge, the boundary object plays an important role in international development, facilitating collaboration among actors with different interests and visions of what development looks like and what development priorities ought to be. "International development" is an increasingly heterogenous field with much internal diversity in stances and agendas—a world in need of boundary objects.

Boundary objects are useful and necessary for collaboration. They're also dangerous. Rigorous discussion and debate about exactly how a solution fits a problem are necessary to tackling the very real, complex, and urgent problems that miracle foods are often believed to solve. By stymying debate and obscuring the political nature of development problems, the miracle crop offers a perilous boundary object.

Notes

1   This statement glosses much debate about quinoa's origins and the politics of origin stories. Domestication stories are always political as they invoke ownership claims.

2   See McDonell (2016) on the ways quinoa's stigmatization and globalization have affected consumption in Andean countries.

3   Note a parallel to the mission of anthropology as originally conceived to save endangered cultures and languages from disappearing.

4   I have not been able to verify who funded the initial creation of the ICUC, but it is clear from the sporadic newsletters of the center that finding sufficient funding was an issue.

5   See McDonell (2019b) on quinoa's discovery in the culinary worlds and its "revalorization" by elite Peruvian chefs.

6   For more on the dissemination of quinoa seeds across the world, see Bazile et al. (2016).

7   An arroba, the most common measure used to buy and sell quinoa in Peru, is equivalent to 11.5 kg. Because Garre is referring to the early 1990s, a time when exchange rates varied drastically from year to year, it is hard to convert 8–10 soles from this time into a US$, but as is clear from the language, his point is that the amount was very small.

8   The story of the trials and travails of the Ancient Harvest entrepreneurs is fascinating. It is well documented in accounts by Thier (2010) and Berson (2014).

9   Over the course of the 1980s, quinoa gained following among different alternative culinary communities in the United States: macrobiotic dieters, vegetarians, and the broader counter cultural cuisine. Quinoa was known both for its nutritional content and for its connection to the "ancient inca," something that comes up in almost every English language quinoa-related article and recipe from this era. Certainly, there is much to unpack about this, but that's for another chapter.

10   Biodiversity competitions have become a common event for development projects in the Andes to promote. Farmers who specialize in selecting crop varieties compete for the best variety and the most varieties, winning small prizes and recognition.

7

What Makes Food Super? The Post-eugenic Promises of Fish Flour and Other Super Powders

Hannah LeBlanc

On June 29, 1962, *Life* Magazine reported on a scientific and humanitarian breakthrough. US government scientists at the Department of Interior were turning "trash fish" into "a powder that is tasteless, odorless, chemically pure and rich in vital animal proteins." When "mixed in stews, vegetable dishes and baking flour," fish protein concentrate (FPC) could provide 2 billion undernourished people with their daily protein and make the United States the "chief benefactor to the world's hungry" ("A Miracle of the Fishes" 1962). Drawing a starker picture of the political economic stakes, one FPC manufacturer told a group of international students at the University of Illinois that the "'have-nots' ... will either find food, or be given food by those who have it, or they will fight to try to take it from those who have it." He succinctly summarized fish flour's appeal: "Cheap fish protein can turn the Red tide in Latin America" (Levin 1960).

Half a century later, a different kind of food powder hit consumer markets. A new start-up called Your Super began selling powder mixes made of "superfoods" such as maca, chia seeds, spirulina, açaí, and lucuma (Crawford 2019). Sold at "premium" prices and wrapped in minimalist brown packaging, Your Super mixes are named for the results they promise: "Forever Beautiful," "Skinny Protein," and "Muscle Power." With products free of Genetically Modified Organisms (GMOs), additives, dairy, gluten, soy, and animal products and sourced from "Africa, Bolivia, Brazil, Finland, Germany, Greece, Japan, Peru, Romania, Spain & Sri Lanka," Your Super suggests that "ancient" cultures can be the benefactors of overfed but undernourished Americans.

What do these two food powders have to do with one another? On their face, they are fifty years and a world apart. Fish flour sold for pennies per pound;

Your Super powders go for dollars per ounce. Proponents of fish flour touted its scientific origins and reliance on industrial technology; Your Super sells its powders as natural and ancient. Fish flour was designed as a food supplement for poor people in the then-called Third World; Your Super's prices are aimed at wealthier customers, most of whom are in the United States.

Yet, I argue, the makers of fish flour and Your Super operate under the same fundamental assumption. Proponents of fish flour and superfoods aim to transform eaters' bodies and, by extension, their capabilities and the social and economic possibilities open to them. Each seeks biological *and* social improvement through targeted nutritional interventions—the addition of powders to existing foods—in ways that respond to the specific economic and cultural needs of their times. And despite the differences between those times, fish flour and Your Super assume similar bodily hierarchies, hierarchies that also animated American eugenic schemes earlier in the twentieth century.

Your Super and fish flour are useful case studies because they both exemplify larger trends in dietary intervention. Your Super is only one player in an increasingly crowded field of contemporary superfood purveyors. I use Your Super not to call out this particular company's practices, but because it represents this larger field. Your Super powders were born after the contemporary obsession with superfoods was well under way and is thus not an effort to rebrand an existing product (see Reisman, this volume, on the rebranding of existing products as superfoods), but an attempt to take advantage of an established trend. Moreover, Your Super's strategy has been, at least according to their own materials, a smash success: the company reports 1000 percent growth in the past year (Crawford 2019). Fish flour was itself one of several attempts in the 1950s and 1960s by food technologists and nutrition experts to develop high-protein food additives primarily for use in the Third World. Although superfoods and fish flour traverse international borders, my sources speak to the ways each of these powdery comestibles embodied the aspirations and anxieties of their American proponents.

Fish flour, never termed a "super" or functional food in its own time, offers a case study and comparison for today's superfoods, highlighting both the historical contingency of what makes a food "super" and continuities across distinct biopolitical projects. The distance traveled from fish flour to superfood powders traces changes in American consumers' relationships to global markets and nutrition experts. It tracks political economic shifts typically shorthanded as neoliberal: from state-sponsored, population-focused interventions to individuals taking responsibility for their bodily improvement through markets. Both, however, rely on powders to overcome vast distances and to change consumption without changing food systems. Both demonstrate the same obsessive desire to use food powders to make certain kinds of bodies and subjects.

#YourSuper

Your Super began in 2015 as a primarily direct-to-consumer, ecommerce start-up. Like other start-ups, Your Super has a "very good story behind it" (see Guthman, this volume). According to interviews, co-founders Kristen de Groot and Michael Kuech met in business school, when they were professional tennis players. De Groot introduced Kuech to homemade "superfood" mixes after he was diagnosed with cancer in his twenties (Boyd 2018). Since the company's founding, it has raised $7.5 million in funding and has reached 500,000 customers, 60 percent of whom, according to Your Super's own data, had never eaten a superfood before buying the company's mixes (Crawford 2019).

Although Your Super avoids explicit health claims, its website implicitly presents its mixes as a remedy for larger structural problems in the American health and food systems. The company reports that 70 percent of their customers are not from urban areas—"they are from the middle of the country in the US where they don't have Whole Foods"—and that a quarter of their customers "have a pre-existing health condition that could benefit from a healthy approach to eating" (Crawford 2019). According to Your Super's website, nine out of ten people do not eat enough fruits and vegetables. These statistics suggest that Your Super products fill a gap in the fresh food market and have health benefits for people with "pre-existing health conditions." The founders' own athletic bodies, featured extensively on their website and Instagram account, are part of the sales pitch. More directly, Kuech recounts his own story of using superfoods while recovering from cancer, and many customer testimonials on the company's website also make stronger health claims for the products. One customer writes that superfoods, together with homeopathy and immunotherapy, helped him recover from stage 4 lung cancer. Others report less remarkable but still impressive benefits: radiant skin, weight loss, better mood, mental clarity, and the feeling of "life flowing through my body" ("Happy Customers" n.d.). Your Super is similarly grandiose in the beneficial results they claim of their products. It sells seven mixes—Muscle Power, Power Matcha, Energy Bomb, Chocolate Lover, Forever Beautiful, Super Green, and

Skinny Protein—which are described as providing "Immunity," "Focus & Brain Power," "Natural Energy," weight loss, clear skin, and relaxation.

In contrasting its product to industrial food, Your Super also taps into fears about the untrustworthiness of supply chains and government regulation. In interviews, the founders emphasize the challenges of ensuring a safe and ethical supply chain. De Groot says:

> One of [our] biggest challenges was learning about corruption in supply chains. It was like, 'Ok how does it work? Where does it come from? Do you test every batch?' … If I don't feel comfortable eating my own products, what's the point in even creating them? So we made a very conscious decision to be a more premium brand, and to source only the best ingredients. We have accurate third party tests on every batch.
>
> (Molvar 2018)

Each product includes a barrage of labels indicating its purity: certified organic, non-GMO, 100 percent plant-based, and gluten-, additive-, dairy-, sweetener-, and soy-free. The purity and "naturalness" of these powders are, ironically, guaranteed by their industrial processing (Smith-Howard 2013). As Loyer (2016c, 168) points out, a powder sprinkled on a smoothie is by definition not whole and unprocessed.

Despite the necessary processing, Your Super draws on a language of naturalness, ancientness, and indigeneity to promote their foods as super. Baobab fruit and guarana sourced from Brazil, chia seeds from Nicaragua, maca root from Peru, and wheatgrass from Germany promise a higher density of vitamins, antioxidants, fiber, and protein than can be found in more familiar foods ("Ingredients" n.d.). Kuech writes in the company's newsletter: "*These nutrient-rich natural ingredients have been used for thousands and thousands of years* by indigenous tribes and forgotten civilizations all around the world with incredible results!" ("Everything changed" n.d., emphasis original). Here, superfoods take their authority not from scientific expertise but from "nutritional primitivism" (Loyer 2016a; Loyer and Knight 2018). Their distance (spatial and, thus, chronological) from the company's mostly US-based consumers lends the powders an almost supernatural authority (Helms 1988). Ancient superfoods from faraway places are contrasted with "modern," industrialized foods, which lack something unspecified but essential.[1]

At the same time, Your Super does not jettison scientific authority. Superfood discourse sits uncomfortably with mainstream or hegemonic nutrition (Hayes-

Conroy and Hayes-Conroy 2013). Your Super uses nutrition's language of quantified macro- and micro-nutrients and boasts that its mixes are approved by "holistic nutritionists." But credentialed nutritionists typically disparage the superfood label as meaningless or at best undefined (Nogrady 2016; "Superfoods or Superhype" n.d.). As Loyer (2016b) argues, superfood discourse straddles cultural categories of nature and science, of medicine and food. Your Super uses this ambiguity to its advantage. It taps into many sources of authority—science, nature, and indigeneity—and combines reductionist nutritionism discourses with nutritional primitivism. This ambiguity suggests benefits beyond those company specifically enumerates.

As an e-commerce retailer, Your Super maintains a significant online presence, particularly on Instagram. Your Super's Instagram consists mostly of artistically arranged food sprinkled with colorful powders. The bodies that are present are nearly exclusively light-skinned, thin, able-bodied, athletic, and female (co-founder Kuech is the main exception). While the company's own images do not necessarily reflect their clientele, it suggests the normative bodies the company promotes. The photographs overwhelmingly exclude people of color. The only exceptions are a farmer in a post about supply chains and a child who is singled out as an object of Your Super's charity. These posts discuss the company's transparent supply chain, ethical supply practices, and food donations. These images are used to bolster the company's claims to ethical capitalism, but in neither case are people of color depicted as consumers of Your Super products.

Your Super promises not only nutrient-dense powders, but transparent supply chains, pure ingredients, and ethical labor practices. In discussing the company's supply chains, De Groot said: "We ensure the people who are growing the ingredients, or processing them are treated well and paid fairly," though those practices are never spelled out in more detail (Molvar 2018). Under the headline of "Giving Back," the company touts its partnership with Action Against Hunger to donate food bars for every mix sold, most recently to refugees in Uganda ("Giving Back" n.d.). By combining messages about bodily and ethical purity, Your Super perpetuates the illusion that consumers can extract themselves from ethically compromised, toxic food systems (Hall 2014; Shotwell 2016). As with other superfood products, what makes Your Super's mixes "super" is not only enhanced nutrition, but also the company's claims to a range of social good, whether or not those claims are verifiable (see Guthman and McDonell, this volume).

Plenty of Fish in the Sea

Superfood manufacturers were not the first to discover the wonders of food powders. Dehydration is an old preservation technique, but since the mid-twentieth century, the US military, in concert with food producers, embraced dehydration and pulverization as means to render foods lightweight and shelf stable. In the Second World War, soldiers sipped rehydrated coffee and ate dried eggs; in the Space Age, astronauts rehydrated dried roast beef in space and Tang took the country by storm (Ensminger et al. 1994, 646; Foss 2015, 161, 168; Risch 1953, 183). In the 1950s and 1960s, food technologists in government, academia, and industry used the technology of pulverization to develop high-protein food powders from a variety of different materials.

In most cases, food technologists tried to creatively repurpose industrial byproducts or animal feeds for human consumption. Cottonseeds, oilseeds, peanuts, and soy were turned into edible powders (Carpenter 1994; see Stein, this volume). Dried non-fat milk, which dominated the international aid scene in the 1950s, was itself a byproduct of creameries.[2] Fish flour or FPC was one such high-protein food product. Fish were defatted, dehydrated, and pulverized into an off-white substance.[3] Like other protein supplements, fish flour came out of the animal feed industry, where agriculturalists had been using fish meal as a protein supplement in chicken and livestock feeds. Fish meal was cheap because it was made from what industry specialists called "trash fish": the small, commercially useless fish that would get caught along with more highly prized ones (Carpenter 1994). Fish flour for human consumption differed from fish meal in that it had higher percentage of fat extracted and faced higher hygienic production standards. Technologists hoped to achieve a tasteless fish flour, one that could be snuck into staple foods without consumers' knowledge. If producers were aware of existing dried fish products common to many global foodways, they did not acknowledge them (Hamada and Wilk 2019, 21). They assumed the only acceptable fish powder was an imperceptible one.

By the 1950s, protein had become the international "charismatic nutrient" (Kimura 2013, 19). Nutritionists trace the interest in protein to Cicely Williams's 1932 identification of kwashiorkor (protein deficiency, especially in children) as a distinct form of malnutrition when she was working as a medical officer in the Gold Coast. Williams named the disease, but international interest did not take off until the establishment of the United Nation's Food and Agricultural Organization (FAO) and World Health Organization (WHO) in 1946 and 1948, which organized researchers to identify cases of kwashiorkor throughout Africa

(Ruxin 2000). In 1955, the UN established the Protein Advisory Group (PAG), a body of international nutrition experts dedicated to questions of protein malnutrition. Drawing on data collected with US government sponsorship, the PAG and other international agencies identified the "global protein gap" between rich and poor countries as the world's defining food problem.

The protein gap theory was attractive as a liberal alternative to eugenic theories for population differences that, while formally discredited after Nazi atrocities had come to light, still inflected much First World thinking about the Third World. As historians of American eugenics have argued, eugenic ideas were versatile and continued to influence everything from marriage counseling to genetics long after the term had been abandoned (Kline 2001; Lombardo 2011; Stern 2016). Federico Gómez, a pediatrician and nutrition researcher in Mexico City, demonstrated how nutrition could be used to rethink population difference: because of chronic malnutrition, he wrote, "large groups of the Mexican population appear to be weary, sad, indifferent, without sense of responsibility, without ambition. From the economic viewpoint, they scarcely produce or consume, enduring the nutritional misery of their lives with stoic fatalism." This lassitude and economic backwardness were not, according to Gómez, inherent: "Those who examine superficially these human groups may attribute their condition to racial traits, considering them lazy, filthy, fatalistic and with no ambition in life. Frequently, observers are not aware that these people are sick" (1961). Nutrition science made this pejorative description of an entire nation palatable to experts and government officials in this post-eugenics moment. Mexicans' supposed faults could be chalked up to their diet rather than to some permanent dimension of their character. International nutritionists drew on Gómez's and others' research on early childhood malnutrition and learning deficits to argue that malnutrition was a cornerstone in cycles of poverty and underdevelopment (Cravioto et al. 1966; Culley 1975; Scrimshaw and Gordon 1968). While Gómez here discusses malnutrition broadly, protein continued to be identified as the most important nutrient in development, and Gómez himself experimented with and promoted fish flour.

Racial and national improvement through dietary reform was not new. Meat, as well as wheat, had long been seen in Anglo-American circles as a driver of their supposed racial and imperial superiority (Veit 2015, 105). Jeffrey Pilcher shows that Mexican elites tried (and failed) to make wheat the center of a national Mexican cuisine, attacking corn as nutritionally inferior and thus unable to support national development (1998, 3, 77–97).[4] But fish flour and other protein supplements offered a new twist: racial improvement without cultural reform or significant dietary change. By taking advantage of industrial food processing techniques, fish flour promised to raise protein (and thus development) without having to alter stubborn dietary habits.

After the Second World War, with the nominal demise of eugenics, nutritional explanations held new appeal for Americans thinking about the Third World.[5] Moreover, nutrition provided a means to frame bodily difference in ways consistent with increasingly dominant modernization theory. American adherents to modernization theory posited a common track of development, from "traditional" societies to "modern" ones, entailing shifts in governmental, economic, and social structures. As historians of modernization theory have shown, while formally detached from time or place, "modern" in this view typically resembled what American liberals hoped for their country (Cullather 2010, 76; Gilman 2003; Latham 2000). Modern nations, according to these theorists, had government-supported industries, progressive tax systems, and substantial social benefits. They were technologically sophisticated, economically advanced, and democratic. They celebrated science and were guided by experts. According to the protein gap theory, the diets of developing countries should also mimic American ones, at least in nutritional content.

By 1960, protein had not only become the central charismatic nutrient in international circles; it was increasingly seen as a potential weapon in the Cold War. In international nutritionists' thinking, better nutrition—especially protein nutrition—would increase human efficiency and help drive a virtuous cycle toward free market capitalism and democracy. This is how fish flour proponents could claim: "Cheap fish protein can turn the Red tide in Latin America" and elsewhere. Providing protein for the whole world, however, posed problems. While international nutritionists were formulating the "protein gap" theory, other thinkers were describing ecological limits to growth. Popularized in 1968 by biologist Paul Ehrlich as the "population bomb," American intellectuals predicted that with unchecked population growth the world would run out of food by the end of the century. Protein, in the animal form most popular in the United States, required especially large amounts of land to produce. In the 1945 book, *The World's Hunger*, Frank Pearson and Floyd Harper predicted the earth could only support 3 billion people at an "Asiatic" standard with little meat and less than a billion at the meat-heavy North American standard (Belasco 2006).

The simultaneous anxieties about the protein gap and population bomb explain fish flour's popularity among policymakers: high-protein powders promised to elevate Third World protein levels without the ecological costs of raising meat.

As an animal protein, fish flour was more appealing to nutrition experts than competing protein foods sourced from plants. To fish flour proponents, the sea seemed to be an escape valve, a near-infinite, self-replenishing source of high-quality animal protein that used no precious arable soil. Nutrition experts imagined that high-protein additives could boost the protein content of diets around the world without having to fundamentally change culinary practices; they would be imperceptible additives in existing foods. As McDonell has argued about the depiction of quinoa as a "miracle crop," this understanding of global malnutrition "depoliticize[s] hunger through a 'curative metaphor'" (McDonell 2015; Kimura 5). Fish flour would be such a cure, not only for hunger but also for economic underdevelopment and even the temptations of communism.

In the United States, one of the first drivers of fish flour was biochemist Ezra Levin, who ran a small pharmaceutical company called VioBin. He understood from the beginning that fish flour would hold great appeal for Cold War nutrition policymakers and began a campaign to build support for the idea and find scientific evidence for its wholesomeness and usefulness. Levin donated samples to researchers working in Mexico, El Salvador, Venezuela, Indonesia, India, and South Africa in the late 1950s. Gómez, the doctor quoted lamenting Mexicans' "nutritional misery" above, became a particularly enthusiastic collaborator (Gómez 1961). The audience of these trials was not future consumers of fish flour, but the politicians who might support government programs to purchase and distribute large quantities of the substance. Despite the feeding trials, most international experts were unimpressed with VioBin's results. VioBin was the only company producing fish flour on a large scale, but the manufacturing process was too inconsistent and used a solvent that many feared might leave toxic residues ("A Satisfactory Process" 1961).

Scientists at the Bureau of Commercial Fisheries (BCF), part of the US Department of the Interior, were intrigued by fish protein powder. The Department of the Interior was led by one of the youngest members of Kennedy's cabinet, Stewart Udall, who encouraged the department to embrace Kennedy's "new frontier" ethos of applying scientific ingenuity to solve social problems (Pariser et al. 1978, 22). Moreover, incomes for commercial fishery workers were dropping relative to the rest of the country, and their numbers were declining ("Needs, goals, and objectives" 1967). The BCF saw an opportunity to do "with fishery resources, what USDA has done in developing such new products as defatted peanuts, orange juice concentrate, instant potato flakes, grapefruit powder, instant applesauce, stabilized soy bean salad oil, nonfat dry milk and freeze-dried foods," which is to say, reinvigorate the industry by developing new fish products, especially shelf-stable ones ("Accelerated Food from the Sea Program" 1967, 5–6). The bureau proposed an ambitious research and development program starting in 1961 to develop fish flour.

By 1966, the BCF had spent $1,740,500 developing FPC, a name they chose to distance their product from Levin's, as well as clarify that it could not replace wheat flour ("Information Requested" 1966). The BCF was optimistic about its new product, estimating that eventually 1 million people would consume 10 grams a day in the United States alone. To fulfill this projected need, the country would require 11 tons of FPC daily, requiring two plants processing 24,000 tons of fish a year, which would give an annual $1,620,000 boost to the fish industry ("Fish Protein Concentrate" 1966). Whereas quality farmland was a highly scarce resource, the BCF treated the seas as nearly limitless, estimating that 200–250 million tons of fish could be removed each year while still following good conservation practices (Butler and Holston 1966).

Fish flour was soon picked up by the US AID Food for Peace program. In the fall of 1967, the agency proposed a major "food from the sea" program, with 42 million dollars over five years dedicated to fish protein alone ("Accelerated Food from the Sea Program" 1967). The agency began surveying Latin American and Asian countries as possible homes for a new demonstration fish flour plant (Food from the Sea Service 1967). Humanitarian reasoning dovetailed with strategic and business interests. Indonesia and Malaysia were particularly attractive because fish flour would be the first and only US aid to the country and thus provided "an unusual opportunity ... for the U.S. to reap political benefits from FPC assistance." However, it might risk "a propagandistic label" if done unilaterally ("Report of Subcommittee" 1967, 7). Although neither Indonesia nor Malaysia was chosen, the State Department did use fish flour as a bargaining chip. Peru and Ecuador were rejected as sites for fish flour experiments in retaliation for detaining and fining US tuna clippers in their waters, or, as a confidential AID planning memo put it, for "rigid adherence to excessive extension of offshore fishing limits" (Pariser et al. 1978, 48; "Report of Subcommittee" 1967; "U.S. State Department" 1967). One of the criteria for selecting recipients of FPC was "Opportunities for furthering U.S.-foreign policy objectives" ("Conversation with Dr. Weinberg" 1967).

Despite their mutual support for the fish flour project, BCF and AID were at odds: the BCF hoped fish flour would bolster American fisheries; AID expected developing nations to open plants in a program that would emphasize "self-help." As McDonell demonstrates with ongoing debates about quinoa as a supercrop (this volume), fish flour served as a "boundary object" for these different US government agencies: they agreed in principle that fish flour was a food with benefits both nutritional and economic, but disagreed about who should benefit and in what ways. The governments requesting technical aid in feeding projects had their own ideas about fish flour's benefits as well.

A series of events conspired to end the fish flour project just as it was getting started. The company AID had contracted to produce fish flour struggled to find enough hake to churn up. The plant had poor quality control as well: of the 1,000 tons ordered, AID deemed only 139 acceptable (most of this went to Chile, which rejected it as inferior to its own product). By 1970, with the fiscally conservative Nixon administration in power and AID's Office of War on Hunger closed, AID began to shutter the fish flour program. At the same time, the BCF program continued to struggle to produce fish flour under insufficient appropriations. When it finally got its demonstration plant off the ground in March of 1971, it ran for just over a year. In that time it produced only 47.3 tons of fish flour that met Food and Drug Administration (FDA) specifications. The product cost more than predicted (over 5 dollars a pound, as opposed to the expected 35–50 cents) and required more fish than predicted. The BCF had also vastly overestimated fish supplies: hake and menhaden, the two FDA-approved sources, were already overfished (Pariser et al. 1978, 50–70, 158). The bill to authorize another $1.3 million for the program never left committee (Comptroller General of the United States 1973).

By the early 1970s, the protein gap theory had also come under attack. In the 1960s, nutritionists had begun referring to "protein-calorie malnutrition," a vague term meant to capture a larger spectrum of malnourishment than protein malnutrition alone (McLaren 1966). Despite the addition of "calorie," most international focus remained on the "impending protein crisis" into the 1970s (United Nations 1971). The major blow fell in 1974, when Donald McLaren, a nutritionist at the American University in Beirut, published a forceful denunciation of the "Great Protein Fiasco" in *The Lancet* (McLaren 1974). Building on earlier critiques (McLaren 1966), he argued that nutritionists had incorrectly extrapolated from cases of kwashiorkor they had encountered in Africa to the rest of the world. For most, he argued, the solution was not more protein but more food. McLaren also took issue with nutritionists' faith that they could solve global hunger with protein powders; he pointed out that most were beyond poor people's incomes, and the ones that had been successful commercially were used as soft drinks or pet food. The fish flour experiment was over.

Was Fish Flour a Superfood?

Was fish flour a superfood? On the face of it, no: the term is anachronistic. Moreover, fish flour, with its reductionist logic, shares more traits with functional foods than today's superfoods (see Spackman, this volume). Yet, though it was never called a "superfood," proponents hoped fish flour would be come a super food. As other contributors to this volume have suggested, superfoods are super because they claim to go above and beyond the nourishment of bodies: they can also help alleviate poverty, solve malnutrition, mitigate climate change and deforestation, and produce "superhuman" subjects (see Guthman; Stein; McDonell; Reisman, this volume).

Fish flour and Your Super are defined as super in different ways. Like other food fortification projects, makers of fish flour and superfood powders propose technological fixes to social and political problems (Rosner 2004). The ambitions of each powder's proponents respond to their political and cultural moments. Fish flour and Your Super represent two different poles of biopower—collective intervention and individual subjectification (Foucault 1990 [1978], 139, Rabinow and Rose 2006). Fish flour was meant to act directly on Third World bodies: its concentrated protein would shake Third World populations out of their lassitude and "nutritional misery"—though the mechanism for such a dramatic change remained vague. This targeted technological intervention was meant to ripple through economic and political structures, pushing Third World countries down the path of modernization. Fish flour was at once dietary intervention, technical assistance, development project, and Cold War weapon. Your Super, conversely, works on individual bodies through the market. Its powders promise to make consumers "superhuman," providing the edge they need to succeed in a competitive world (see Reisman, this volume; Sikka 2017, 87–107). At the same time, it claims to transform supply chains, improve labor practices, and help end hunger through private philanthropy. Your Super suggests its powders help consumers circumvent failing regulatory systems, toxic foods, and unethical business practices.

The distance between their political and social ambitions is not coincidental: superfood discourse traces historical transformations that are reflected in food politics more broadly. Your Super represents a partial consumer backlash against the kind of technology and expertise fish flour represented. The company's marketing evinces a skepticism toward food processing, government regulation, health care, and scientific expertise that was born the same moment that fish flour was dying. Controversies over DDT, thalidomide, cyclamate, and fluoridated water undermined confidence in regulatory science and the "universal choiceworthiness" of industrialized food (Bobrow-Strain 2011). Meanwhile, the "counter cuisine" began experimenting with farming, vegetarianism, and macrobiotics (Belasco 2007). The global protein gap was premised in part on the idea that the American diet was one the world should try to emulate, within ecological limits. Superfoods today are premised on the opposite idea: that American diets and food systems are deeply flawed; that Americans must look to faraway peoples and places untinged with modernity to rescue their health. And although protein has once again become a national charismatic nutrient, meat has become one of the most controversial dimensions of the American diet. Fish flour proponents touted the fact that their product contained only superior animal protein; Your Super boasts that their protein powders are animal-free.

Despite the distance traveled, these two powders share fundamental assumptions. Today's superfoods are implicated in a longer lineage of biopolitical projects that seek to transform populations through individual bodily intervention, a lineage that includes eugenics. Fish flour's popularity depended on the turn to nutrition to explain and solve perceived national problems in the wake of the Second World War. Like eugenicists, fish flour proponents argued bodily transformation was central to social and economic improvement. More significantly, they also maintained eugenicists' ideas about which bodies were most admirable and which lives most deserving. Today's superfood projects make these hierarchies less explicit, but the expense, the extraction of products from the Global South to the Global North, and the overwhelming whiteness of Your Super's marketing materials imply such a hierarchy nonetheless. In these hierarchies, choice and control over one's diet are a political prerogative guaranteed to those at the top but denied to those at the bottom.

Expanding our view of superfood discourse links the tacit forms of persuasion in contemporary superfood discourse to the longer history of more coercive attempts to control the diets, and lives, of people marginalized by race, geographic location, and body size (Biltekoff 2013; Dupuis 2015; Kimura 2013; Kimura et al. 2014; Moran 2018). Foods that purport to be "super" tie together what is good to eat with what kinds of lives are good to live. While the two powders discussed here offer technical solutions in different political economic circumstances, the kinds of bodies and subjects they seek to create are remarkably similar. These two nutrition interventions discard some of eugenics' most odious characteristics—the focus on heredity, race, and breeding—but they have failed to abandon eugenics' hierarchies of bodies, races, and nations. In the light of such alimentary racism and ableism (Hall 2014; Probyn 2000), such foods appear less super.

Notes

1   Many dietary discourses tap into fears about modern diets. In *Diet and the Disease of Civilization* (2017), Adrienne Rose Bitar argues that this kind of "fall of man" story is a near-universal trope in twentieth-century American diet books.

2   It had been developed by the Farm Chemurgic Council with support from the USDA in the 1920s and 1930s as a response to outrage over the untreated dairy waste that was polluting waterways (Pursell 1969; Smith-Howard 2013).

3   Unless the distinction is important, I used these terms interchangeably. Some also called it Marine Protein Concentrate or Fish Powder, though these names never caught on.

4   As Pilcher points out, Mexican elites used nutritional explanations for racial difference to avoid biological determinist theories. In the United States and Europe, determinist eugenic ideas had long co-existed comfortably with "euthenics" (improvement of the race through diet and hygiene) (Veit 2013).

5   The mania for animal protein infected ecological anthropologists too, who experienced a brief infatuation with "protein determinism," the idea that the need to maximize animal protein drove the development of cultural traits (Diener et al. 1980).

Part Three

Superfood Trajectories

From Superfood to Staple? Tracing the Complex Commoditization of Kale

Marvin Joseph F. Montefrio and Anacorita O. Abasolo

During the late 2000s, kale—a leafy vegetable closely related to broccoli, cauliflower, brussels sprouts, and collard greens—transformed from a humble vegetable into a culinary superstar in the West, particularly the United States. Native to Asia Minor and the Mediterranean, this crop was brought to Northern and Western Europe more than two millennia ago and eventually to North America by the European colonists (Field 2000; Kiple 2000). While kale was once a common vegetable in Northern Europe that peasants produced and consumed (O'Hagan 2019; Sheraton 1976), it eventually fell into obscurity, when compared to its more popular cousins, broccoli and brussels sprouts (Shamsian 2016). In the United States, kale was commonly produced in small-scale farms and household gardens for use as a mere garnish in restaurant dishes (Hanna 2012). This changed after 2010, when Michelin starred and prominent farm-to-table restaurants across the United States began featuring kale prominently in their menus. Around the same time, a number of celebrities, including Gwyneth Paltrow, Ellen DeGeneres, and Dr. Oz, endorsed the green for its dense nutritional content (Quinn 2018; Wilson 2015). With demand growing, kale production in the United States increased dramatically, with the total harvest between 2007 and 2017 increasing almost fourfold (USDA 2014, 2019).

Kale's story of transformation from obscurity to fame in the United States has been widely explored in popular media. Our interest in this chapter, however, is to follow its trajectory in geographic contexts where it was recently introduced as a novel healthy food trend. How does its status as a commodity travel outside the United States or the West? How does its status change over time, following culinary trends taking place locally, in the West, and elsewhere? We explore these questions by examining the case of the Philippines, a Southeast Asian country with vibrant foodways that has adopted the kale trend from the United States in the 2010s.

Kale derives its booming popularity from its marketing as a superfood. Ever since it garnered attention in the Western culinary world, recipe books, social media sites, and food blogs have consistently identified the green as a superfood. Superfoods are often marketed for their healthfulness due to their supposedly elevated phytochemical and micronutrient content, ambiguously straddling the categories of food and medicine (Loyer 2019; Lunn 2006). While superfoods appear to be a critique of the contemporary industrial agri-food system (Loyer and Knight 2018), Loyer (2019) argues that such a "critique is flawed because of the tendency for the values [they promote] to become commodified, as superfood products are produced, marketed, and sold for profit" (p. 2270). She warns that as superfood commodities gain popularity worldwide and become fetishized, their production and consumption may lead to inequitable economic relations that deprive underprivileged and marginalized populations of access to their benefits. Sikka (2017) cautions of the propensity of new foodstuffs branded as superfoods (e.g., those with "exotic" origins such as maca and açaí) to be co-opted by the capitalist agri-food system, and they may become entrenched in unjust commodity chains and controlled by large agri-food businesses and transnational corporations. Meanwhile, familiar food commodities such as almonds are being rebranded as superfoods to allow the agri-food industry to address overproduction and continue capital accumulation (Reisman, this volume).

We argue that binary framings of superfoods as good or bad, critical of or complicit in capitalism, radically oversimplify the complex and varied realities of superfoods. We agree that superfoods are inevitably entrenched in capitalist markets, but we believe they can have complex social lives that are irreducible to "capitalist takeover." The complexity becomes more apparent when we analyze their forms, uses, movements, and trajectories across geographies and time. We follow Appadurai's (1986) conceptualization of a commodity as "not one kind of thing rather than another, but one phase in the life of some things" (p. 17; see also Kopytoff 1986). Hence, it undergoes a process of *commoditization* where it moves in and out of a particular commodity state (e.g., shifting between capitalist and other forms of commodities) in a given phase of a commodity's life. This process is differentiated and it can be "slow or fast, reversible or terminal, normative or deviant" (Appadurai 1986, 13). Not only do commodities shift states; capitalist and other commodity forms can co-exist and incorporate each other's characteristics (Tsing 2013).

Rather than analyzing commodities as dichotomies (e.g., commodities or gifts, or capitalist and non-capitalist),[1] we adopt Jack Manno's (2000, 2002, 2010) concept of *commodity potentials*, which combines Appadurai's commodity state and its candidacy (i.e., the symbolic and classificatory ways of defining the exchangeability of things). Manno depicts a spectrum of commodity states—that is, between high and low commodity potentials—based on a good or service's traits and attributes in a system of exchange. Goods and services with higher commodity potential (e.g., exported comestibles) are highly mobile, transferable, standardized, efficient, and, in many cases, excludable. On the other hand, goods and services with lower commodity potential (e.g., food produced in home gardens) are locally situated, heterogeneous, more complex, focused on social relations, and can be more inclusive and accessible to a wide spectrum of producers and consumers (see McLeod-Kilmurray 2012; Montefrio 2012, for more food examples). The commodity potential of goods and services *may*, in given contexts, indicate whether they are consumed by those of higher-class status (i.e., excludable) or across socioeconomic classes (i.e., inclusive).[2] Between high and low potential is a vast array of commodities susceptible to transformation from low to high or vice versa.

The factors that determine the trajectory of commoditization include, for example, social relations and knowledge production associated with the commodity, as well as the material characteristics and properties of objects (Cook and Crang 1996; Glover and Stone 2018). Knowledge production is of particular interest in commoditization, especially when we take into consideration *credence qualities*. Credence qualities are information on commodities that are presented to consumers through various marketing strategies, the veracity of which is often difficult for consumers to evaluate on their own (Darby and Karni 1973).[3] In the realm of food, typical credence qualities include "organic," "fair trade," "local," "heirloom," and "superfood." These qualities enhance the commodity potential of goods and services by affording premiums to their exchange value (Glover and Stone 2018). The scale and direction of commoditization, however, are contingent and contextual (Appadurai 1986). Hence, superfood commodities, depending on where and when they emerge, may have varying material and discursive manifestations, undergo multidirectional changes, and follow a plethora of possible trajectories.

If we exclusively examine kale's rapid rise in popularity as a superfood commodity in the United States, we might conclude that kale (and all other superfoods) is subject to capture and co-optation by the capitalist agri-food system. Indeed, marketing agencies, celebrities, social media influencers, the culinary industry, and large-scale growers have helped to elevate kale to fame, capturing the palates of privileged classes willing to pay the price. However, following the trajectory of kale beyond the United States reveals that kale's commodity life does not follow the typical "rags to riches" narrative we see in other superfoods such as quinoa (see, for example, McDonell 2015). Focusing on the shifting commodity potentials and associated class status of kale in the Philippines, we demonstrate that kale had high commodity potential, and was adopted through privileged culinary circuits involving large-scale producers, high-end restaurants and markets, manufacturers, and exporters. Its credence quality as a superfood has differentiated it as more valuable than other locally available leafy greens and vegetables in the country. Initially, kale was an excludable, mobile, and standardized high-value commodity in the Philippines. Over time kale with low commodity potential has also emerged in the Philippines. Less privileged Filipinos now grow kale in home gardens and have integrated it into local dishes, and exchanged it through kin and community networks. We argue that the complex interactions between kale's credence qualities and its materiality (i.e., a nutritious hardy crop with close relations to other familiar local Brassicas) have allowed, at least for a time, the co-existence of kale's high and low commodity potentials, reflecting Wilk's (2006) concept of "style sandwich."

Our analysis and findings are based on qualitative fieldwork and discourse analysis of social media posts. We carried out semi-structured, in-depth interviews with thirty kale growers in the island of Luzon in the Philippines who produce kale either as part of a commercial supply chain or for personal consumption (or both); eighteen regular kale consumers; and ten proprietors of retail stores and restaurants who sell kale as a raw vegetable, part of a prepared dish, and/or in manufactured and packaged form. We also conducted observations in farms and gardens, farmers' markets, and restaurants, where we learned how growers, retailers, and consumers discuss and imagine kale's value. We also carried out extensive analysis of social media sites (e.g., Instagram accounts of retailers and restaurants and Facebook accounts of growers), the webpages of companies selling kale in the Philippines, locally circulated food magazines, and newspaper articles.

A Brief History of Vegetables in the Philippines

The Philippines has diverse foodways, owing not just to its archipelagic geography but also to its long history of trade with China, India, and Arabia, and Spanish (1521–1898) and American (1898–1946) colonization (Kirshenblatt-Gimblett and Fernandez 2003, 61). While Filipinos commonly identify foods based on a connection to a specific hometown, province, or region (e.g., *Ilonggo* food from the Panay islands), professional culinary spaces increasingly use the terms "Filipino food" or "Philippine food," promoting the emergence of a national cuisine. Food scholars commonly characterize today's Philippine food as the result of the indigenization of foreign ingredients and cooking styles during the precolonial, colonial, and postcolonial periods (Fernandez and Alegre 1988). Some scholars go so far as to describe Filipinos as having a penchant for any food considered "foreign," in particular those linked to Europe and the United States. Urban Filipinos have always been quick to adopt foreign food trends, such as imported comestibles (e.g., fruits and canned goods introduced during the American colonial regime) and culinary trends from the Euro-Americas (e.g., fast-food chains, third-wave coffee shops, farm-to-table restaurants) (Doeppers 2016; Fernandez 1994; Matejowsky 2009; Montefrio 2020; Montefrio et al. 2020; Palanca 2016).

The diversity of the country's vegetable foodways reflects this culinary mélange. Quite a few of the vegetable dishes that are considered quintessentially Filipino actually exemplify foreign influences. Doeppers (2016), for example, documents how particular crops from the Brassica family that are normally found in the West—for example, cabbage (*Brassica oleracea* var. capitata) and cauliflower (*Brassica oleracea* var. botrytis)—were already grown in the Philippine highlands over a century ago. The Chinese cabbage, pechay (*Brassica rapa pekinensis*), that Chinese traders and immigrants introduced was also documented in the highlands and even in Manila and neighboring lowland provinces in the early twentieth century. These introduced crops eventually found their way into Philippine cuisine, such as the cabbage in *nilagang baka* (beef soup dish) and the pechay in *ginataang tilapia* (tilapia fish cooked with coconut milk). These foreign influences endure as new vegetables, such as kai lan (*Brassica oleracea* var. alboglabra) and the curly, red, and Tuscan varieties of kale in the Brassica family reach the Philippine shores.

While new vegetables have been introduced in the Philippines over the years, vegetables in general remain a small part of the Filipino diet.

Vegetables constitute no more than a fifth of a typical Filipino meal by weight (Maghirang 2006), and the average daily consumption of vegetables among Filipinos is low as well.[4] In 2008, Filipinos consumed 110 grams of vegetables a day, compared to the recommended daily fruit and vegetable intake of 400 grams set by the WHO.[5] However, there appears to be class differentiation in vegetable consumption. Higher-income Filipinos consume more vegetables (particularly the more expensive vegetables grown in the highlands, like carrots and cabbage) than lower socioeconomic classes. We surmise that the class difference will increase, as higher-income Filipinos, particularly in the urban areas, adopt new culinary concepts based on consuming vegetables from the West.

In Manila, in particular, middle- and upper-class Filipinos increasingly consume salads, juices, and smoothies, incorporating Western ideas of "healthy food" that have gained popularity since 2013. Restaurants that market their menus around organic, farm-to-table, and vegetarian/vegan labels have proliferated in the metropolis, alongside other lifestyle trends that promote fitness and weight loss (e.g., yoga and CrossFit along with diets like paleo, ketogenic, and South Beach) (Montefrio 2020; Montefrio et al. 2020). Euro-American-inspired weekend farmers' markets selling natural and organic produce have also flourished, particularly in or near spaces where the middle and upper classes reside (e.g., elite-gated communities and nearby commercial spaces). Furthermore, foods marketed as "superfoods"—such as chia seeds, açaí berries, cacao, and kale—have become omnipresent in organic, farm-to-table, and vegetarian/vegan restaurants.

Kale's High Commodity Potential

Kale's adoption in the Philippines appears to follow its high commodity trajectory in the United States. Nobody in the Philippines, except for a select few who had encountered kale abroad and in social media, knew about this leafy vegetable before the early 2010s, when cosmopolitan Filipinos with high economic, social, and cultural capital began introducing kale to the Philippines. Filipino chefs and restaurateurs acquired the use of kale through culinary tourism and professional meetings that took place domestically or abroad. Return migrants also contributed to the diffusion of ideas and discourses by bringing back their knowledge and encounters with kale. New media played a critical role by connecting local Filipino cosmopolitans with influencers in the

West who promote health and fitness in food blogs and the social media. Kale in turn captured the attention of Filipino social media influencers, established producers, and privileged local consumers.

The credence qualities associated with kale's branding as a superfood were central to its entry into the privileged culinary circuits of the Philippines. Superfood was a burgeoning discourse when kale arrived in Manila. Ingredients such as chia seeds, cacao nibs, and turmeric were offered in upscale restaurants, supermarkets, and specialty food retail stores. In our field research, it was common to hear proponents of kale—be they restaurant owners and employees, retail market sellers, growers, or consumers—discuss kale's nutritional benefits and ability to protect consumers from diseases such as diabetes, coronary heart disease, and cancer. Most marketing promotions, for instance, highlighted the scientific aspects of its nutritional properties, such as its protein, fiber, vitamins, minerals, fatty acids, and other micronutrients.

A small supply of fresh kale combined with high demand among health- and fitness-conscious Filipino cosmopolitans quickly created a very exclusive market. At this time, kale remains prominent in exclusive culinary circuits in the Philippines. Just as in the cosmopolitan cities of the United States, kale has been featured in gourmet restaurants in Manila that specialize in organic, farm-to-table, and vegetarian/vegan food. It has become a popular culinary offering in farm tourism sites and wellness resorts near Manila where metropolitan dwellers go for respite. It has been integrated as one of the main ingredients in salads, juices, smoothies, and other expensive speciality items. For example, a salad bowl with kale for lunch in a farm-to-table restaurant in Manila cost 450 to 600 pesos in early 2019 (~US$8.65 and US$11.55). In comparison, a typical lunch comprising rice, meat, and vegetable in a canteen or a quick-service restaurant cost no more than 200 pesos (~US$3.85). Restaurants serving kale tend to be found in exclusive commercial spaces where corporate executives, foreign expats, and wealthier metropolitans dine. Restaurateurs justify the cost of kale dishes as a product of low supply. One owner of a healthy juicing bar explained: "Some of our customers complain about why [kale juices] are so expensive. Well, because it is hard to find! You won't be able to buy kale just anywhere … and it is expensive! I know there are already some parts of the Philippines where they grow kale, but sometimes we still import."

Raw kale sold in markets in Manila is expensive. In early 2019, for example, we noted that organic curly and Tuscan kale cost 1000 pesos/kilo (~US$19.25/kilo) and the non-organic varieties were 600 pesos/kilo (~US$11.55/kilo) in an online retail platform. In contrast, the other vegetables of the Brassica family were priced much lower. Organic pechay was sold in the same online retail platform for 360 pesos/kilo (~US$6.95/kilo), cabbage for 350 pesos/kilo (US$6.75/kilo), and broccoli for 580 pesos/kilo (~US$11.15/kilo). This dramatic price difference makes kale the most expensive vegetable in almost every marketplace we visited. In spite and because of the steep price, many consumers still scramble to buy kale.

While kale production remains low, farmers and culinary entrepreneurs increasingly see a business opportunity. Established organic farmers were the first to grow kale commercially in the early 2010s, in anticipation of high returns. As one large-scale organic farmer said, "It's one of the ingredients for vegetable juicing. Isn't juicing the in thing now? That's why I thought kale would sell because they use it for juicing." Another entrepreneur said, "Celebrities are now endorsing that. They say it is a fat burner. That's why it is good to plant that." Some also referred to its credence qualities as a superfood. After explaining in detail the value of kale as a healthy vegetable and a superfood, one entrepreneur admitted, "It is a good business. We sell it in a [farmer's market in Manila] where it has a good market. We are also able to deliver to people who would want to have their own kale. We also sell it in our own retail store. It is really a good business."

Small farmers have also been inspired to get into the kale business. They see kale as a lucrative crop compared to other vegetables. In 2015, we observed a training seminar in an established agritourism organic farm where we witnessed aspiring small organic farmers excited with the new crops they encountered for the first time, like arugula and kale. At the end of the training seminar, several participants bought kale seeds from the farm's souvenir shop. One participant said, "I want the kale (he pronounced it as kah-le). That costs high per kilogram right? Many people buy that, right?" Individual entrepreneurs and established produce consolidators (wholesalers) who bridge farmers and consumers encourage small farmers to grow and introduce kale into existing vegetable supply chains. These middle entities sell the idea to farmers by highlighting the burgeoning popularity of the vegetable in Manila. Farmers are then enticed by the promise of a profitable market. We also observed that a few larger, well-financed farms already growing kale were incorporating small farmers as contract growers into their existing kale supply chain.

The seeds industry has caught up with the trend as well. Local commercial seed companies in the Philippines now sell seeds of curly, red, and Tuscan kale.

Small farmers and growers, however, find these seeds expensive. For example, one small-scale urban farmer explained,

> Kale seeds are expensive, especially compared to vegetables like pechay. For example, if I buy the seeds from the store, the price is all 59 pesos, but if you open the packet of pechay, the seeds are in the thousands. But that's just 59 pesos. If you compare it with kale, also 59 pesos per packet, but only 20 seeds inside. That's why when I go to the store to buy kale seeds, I only get one packet because it is more expensive.

We noticed that farmers and growers tend to focus on curly, red, and Tuscan kale, though its close relative kai lan (also referred to as Chinese broccoli or Chinese kale) has been grown longer and is more abundant. While kai lan is mostly found in upscale farmers' markets and supermarkets, it costs much less than curly, red, and Tuscan kale. Kai lan is not branded as a superfood and many farmers are aware that kale and kai lan all belong to the same species. One farmer explained that he prefers to grow and market curly, red, and Tuscan kale, even if kai lan has its benefits in the consumer standpoint:

> More or less kai-lan is the same as Tuscan and curly kale. For me the taste is the same, but [kai-lan] is leafier per kilo of the vegetable. It is also just 150 pesos a kilo! … but I am very careful. If I educate my consumers about that, there goes the business! [laughs] … Let the people who want to waste their money enjoy their life wasting their money. Well, they don't complain!

Entrepreneurs have not only taken advantage of the value of curly, red, and Tuscan kale; they have also added value by going beyond producing raw vegetables. They have anticipated that there will eventually be a glut in the kale market and that prices will fall. One large-scale kale grower explained:

> Kale is becoming so popular now that sometimes it becomes a challenge because now you have competition […] so we started out with planting kale, but in terms of business you don't get your [return on investment] so much because it is not value added. Then competition comes in, they are not organic, they sell half your price, and then you have a problem.

She had decided to get into manufacturing and invested in machinery to produce instant powdered beverage drinks using the kale they grow. Another team of entrepreneurs began producing kale chips. Their business has since expanded to include kale energy bars and now they export their products to Singapore and Hong Kong.

Kale's Low Commodity Potential

Kale's high commodity state remains vibrant in privileged culinary circuits, but its low commodity potential has also emerged. Lower-income households without capital to spend on pricey organic kale in farmers' markets or kale dishes in organic or farm-to-table restaurants are growing the vegetable for their own consumption. Home growers are independent (i.e., not integrated in established commercial supply chains) and produce kale in relatively small quantities. They still consider kale a superfood, employing the same nutritional discourses about kale that upscale consumers use.

One notable network of independent home growers is the urban farming movement. We recently chanced upon a group of urban gardeners who grow their own vegetables in small containers in whatever limited space their homes can afford. While we met several home growers who attempted to grow curly, red, and Tuscan kale but failed, quite a few have become successful growing these varieties alongside other leafy green vegetables and herbs. A good example is Mr. Bernal, an urban backyard grower who decided to grow organic vegetables at home after realizing that he could not afford to shift to the predominantly plant-based diet that his medical condition requires. In the process of learning about organic food production, he encountered kale and learned to grow curly, red, and Tuscan varieties in his small backyard in Manila. He explained how kale is a hardy crop that can be cultivated in the Philippine lowlands:

> You do need to have a rich soil, because kale needs a lot of nutrients to support its growth. But I did not have any problems with the weather. Even if it is in the cool season or summer I am able to grow kale in a warm place like Manila. It is not like other vegetables [which later on he identified as highland crops like broccoli, cabbage, and carrots] that have a hard time [adapting] to the lowlands. Kale, in my experience, is not too sensitive to the weather.

Urban kale growers obtain information on the crop's nutritional and health benefits and how to grow it from the internet, through blogs, YouTube clips, and conversation with other home growers in Facebook groups. Many of the growers we interviewed are members of a Facebook community of tens of thousands of urban organic gardeners in the Philippines. In this community, they learn to grow kale in limited spaces using recycled materials (e.g., used PET bottles and biscuit containers) and make their own organic fertilizers and pesticides. A few have also learned to successfully save their seeds for the future, relying less on commercial kale seeds in the market. Mr. Bernal, for example, said he is able to keep seeds from his mature kale plants for the next planting cycle. He explained, "I always leave one or two that I allow to mature so I can collect seeds so that I do not need to buy seeds anymore."

Sharing is a common feature in the home growing of kale. Urban growers produce kale for self-consumption and their surplus is either given away to family members or neighbors, or sold at a price significantly lower than in the supermarkets or farmers' markets. One home grower, Ms. Suarez, explained that she gives away some of her harvests and sells kale seedlings at a low price. She said,

> I give my extra harvests away to my friends ... I also sell kale seedlings for 25 pesos [~0.50 USD], which are ready to harvest in a few days. I know the amount I charge is too low, but I treat it almost like a giveaway. I have a friend who said, "why are you selling it too cheap? That's expensive in Manila!", but I said that's okay.

Some share seeds they keep in the hope of encouraging others to plant. One urban kale grower, Ms. Roman, said, "I intend to produce more, so that I can help more, because there are so many people who need the nutrients from kale ... I share my seeds with people I know, hoping that they share with others too. I really believe in sharing the seeds."

The involvement of home growers in the production of kale has also helped facilitate the gradual introduction of this leafy green into everyday Philippine cuisine. Since most Filipinos cannot access kale in its "high commodity" form (e.g., as mixed in salads and smoothies sold in high-end restaurants or in manufactured food products sold in specialty retail stores), home growers have explored ways to prepare kale in their home kitchens. While they have learned to consume kale in American-style salads and juices, they have incorporated kale in creative ways in a number of Philippine dishes that typically use other leafy greens such as pechay, mustard leaves, cabbage, moringa, and taro. Examples include *nilagang baka*, *tinolang manok* (Filipino chicken soup), *pinikpikan* (beaten chicken stew), and *laing* (taro leaves cooked in coconut milk). This practice resonates with Wilk's (2006) notion of substitution in which a typical ingredient in a dish is replaced with something new for various reasons, including the use of a more nutritious or higher-status ingredient. Many home growers we interviewed mentioned that they use curly kale as substitute for pechay because the taste of the former reminds them of the latter. One urban kale grower said:

Table 8.1 Summary of Kale with high and low commodity potentials

	Kale's High Commodity Potential	Kale's Low Commodity Potential
Production	In established production sites primarily for commercial purposes Depends on commercial inputs, some of which are imported such as the seeds	In household gardens and urban backyards and allotments Does not depend on external supply chains; home growers make their own inputs and can keep seeds for future production
	Transformed into high-value commodities, such as manufactured kale products with value addition (kale chips and power bars)	Kept as a raw vegetable, prepared as an ingredient for home cooking
Consumption	Sold in high-end retail stores and gourmet restaurants, particularly to middle- and upper-class consumers	Consumed by the producers themselves and shared (or sold at a very low price) within the producers' immediate community
	Prepared as ingredient in expensive Western dishes	Experimented in everyday Filipino dishes

You can mix [kale] in *nilagang baka* or *tinola*. You can use kale in whatever dishes you cook with pechay. If you compare, kale is tougher so you have to cook it longer to become soft. It is not like pechay that cooks much quickly … you really have to experiment. I, myself, have experimented a lot with kale … I also learn a lot from others I chat with in our FB group.

Our observations point to a simultaneous duality in ways of consuming kale, one with high commodity potential and another with low commodity potential. Table 8.1 provides a summary description of the traits of kale as high and low commodity in production and consumption. We discuss next what this duality means in our understanding of commoditization of superfoods.

Conclusion: Kale's Complex Commoditization

We have demonstrated the complex commoditization of kale in particular, with relevance to superfoods in general. Historically, kale had been produced and consumed with low commodity potential in Western Europe and North America. Only in the last ten years has the leafy green been elevated to culinary prominence in the West and introduced in the Philippines as a high-status commodity through privileged circuits of production and consumption. It has high commodity potential because it is primarily produced for commercial sale; its credence qualities as a superfood allow its advocates to command a high price in the market; its high-value manufactured forms (e.g., kale chips) allow reach to distant markets; it has developed complex and extended supply chains that create dependence on commercial inputs and contracted labor; and finally it is excludable because its steep price rules out the majority of Filipinos from eating it.

We avoided framing the development of kale in the Philippines as merely a narrative of "superfoods captured by the capitalist agri-food system." Instead, we underscore the propensity of superfoods to shift commodity states from high to low and vice versa, and for various commodity forms to co-exist at the same moment (Appadurai 1986; Tsing 2013). As we have shown in this chapter, kale's low commodity potential has emerged and co-existed alongside its high commodity potential in the Philippines. Just a few years after being introduced as a high-value commodity for the elite, kale is now produced for self-sustenance and is shared widely among kin networks for free or within non-monetized exchange and gift networks, or sold at a very low price. Most importantly, Filipinos from the lower classes are now consuming kale in culinary forms that are integrated in everyday Philippine foodways.

How did the low commodity state of kale emerge in the Philippines, given that this vegetable was introduced to Filipinos exclusively through privileged circuits? We point to the complex interplay between the credence qualities of kale and its materiality as a hardy Brassica crop. Following Glover and Stone (2018), the credence qualities of kale as a superfood have indeed contributed to the diffusion of its high commodity forms in the Philippines, framing the leafy green as nutritionally superior to other vegetables. However, the same credence qualities have appealed to consumers from the lower socioeconomic class, as partly explained by the tendency of Filipinos to be open to Western cultural trends. On the other hand, the materiality of kale—its qualities as a plant that can be adapted from temperate to tropical regions—has allowed home growers to develop its low commodity potential. In comparison, other Brassica crops like broccoli and cauliflower that can only grow in the Philippine highlands have sustained their high commodity state for many decades. Furthermore, kale's close relations to Brassica crops common in the Philippines have allowed experimentation and the leafy green's inclusion in mainstream Philippine foodways.

It is still too early to say what the co-existence of high and low commodity potential kale will mean in the future of the leafy green in the Philippines. The emergence of low commodity potential kale has not yet undermined its credence quality as a superfood and its associated class distinction, and the upper class continues to consume and patronize it for its supposed health and nutritional benefits. The production of kale's low commodity form is still much less than its high commodity counterpart. If kale's low commodity potential expands further and/or its superfood status diminishes, perhaps it could become a banal staple just like its relatives that are consumed by both the rich and poor on a daily basis. This trajectory would follow many other foodstuffs like sugar and wheat that have entered the mainstream (Doeppers 2016; Mintz 1985). We see signs of this in the gradual fall of the price of kale in some markets. The other possible trajectory is that kale might just become obscure in the Philippines, as it gets overshadowed by other newly introduced crops or widely available local vegetables that are elevated because of their high-nutritional and health value. This trajectory is plausible given the presence of a coalition of culinary professionals, social enterprises, and nonprofit organizations in the Philippines advocating for "local superfoods" like malabar spinach, sweet potato leaves, and moringa. These could supersede kale one day, especially if they become popular in the West. We emphasize, however, that the eventual fate of superfood kale remains to be seen.

Notes

1   Anna Tsing makes a distinction between commodities and non-commodities (e.g., gifts), following Marx ([1887] 1990). However, we take Appadurai's (1986) position that all things that are exchanged are commodities.

2   Manno does not fully develop the conceptual link between commodity potential and class distinction, although he does say that high commodity potential goods and services may exclude marginalized populations. We do recognize that the link between commodity potential and class distinction is complex. For example, localized commodities (e.g., artisanal products and community-supported agriculture) can be excludable as well. Nonetheless, Manno's typology holds for many commodities and contexts, such as kale in the Philippines.

3   Credence qualities usually require a system that acts as a proxy to consumer evaluation, such as process standards, traceability measures, and certification (Reardon et al. 1999). Appadurai (1986) also alludes to the idea of credence quality in his discussion of knowledge and commodities.

4   According to Maghirang (2006), the average food consumption per capita in the Philippines in 2003 was 879 grams per day, a third of which is rice, a fifth meat, fish, and poultry, and about 14 percent vegetables.

5   https://news.abs-cbn.com/lifestyle/07/04/12/why-pinoys-are-not-eating-their-veggies

9

The Global Açaí: A Chronicle of Possibilities and Predicaments of an Amazonian Superfood

Eduardo S. Brondizio

Introduction

From its origin myth[1] as a salvation food to its regional expansion as a low-income staple to its fame as antioxidant-rich status symbol in the hands of global celebrities, the story of açaí fruit[2] embodies multiple narratives of the superfood. More than a superfood, however, the açaí palm is considered a tree of life and a miracle-plant in its region of origin. Today, the açaí palm defines the landscape along the Amazonian floodplains and increasingly the hinterlands as well. To rural and urban residents alike, the gracious açaí palm is a metonym of place, pride, and identity celebrated in songs and poems, paintings, objects, toys, religious events, local festivals, and in government and corporate advertising (Figure 9.1a). In the Amazon estuary-delta region, residents use the açaí palm in over twenty-five different ways.[3] Unknown outside of the Amazon region until the 1990s, açaí consumption has become ubiquitous in Brazil today and increasingly a symbol of the Amazon and Brazil across the globe (Brondizio 2008).

The presence of açaí fruit in Amazonian life dates back millennia. During the last four decades, a complex regional economy has evolved accompanied by the expansion and intensification of production; multiple types of commodity supply chains; and new nutritional, cosmetic, and pharmaceutical industries, all of which have transformed a humble regional fruit into an international household name. As açaí has gained economic importance in the region, it has

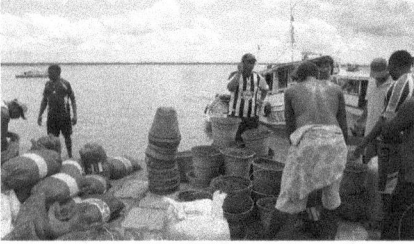

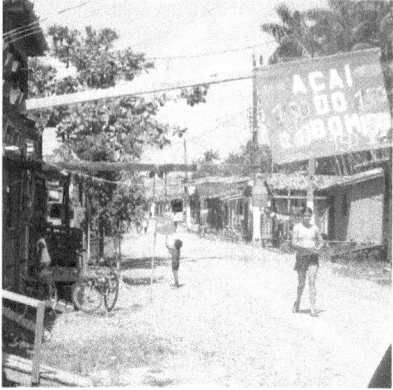

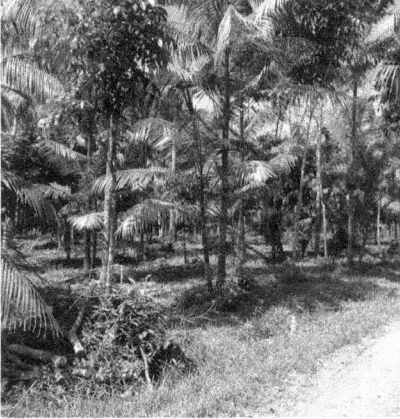

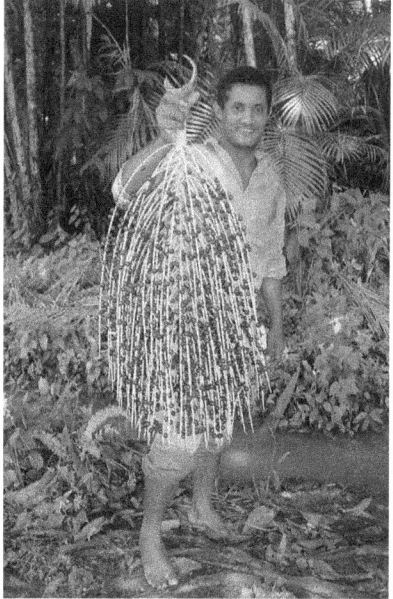

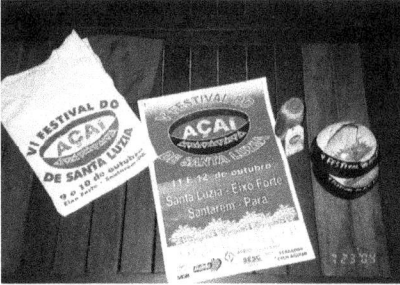

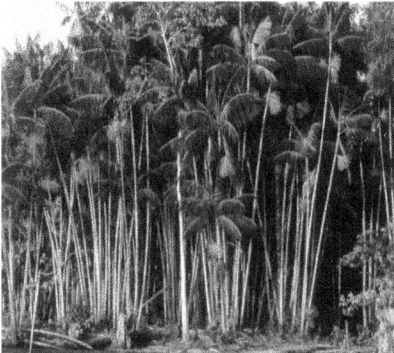

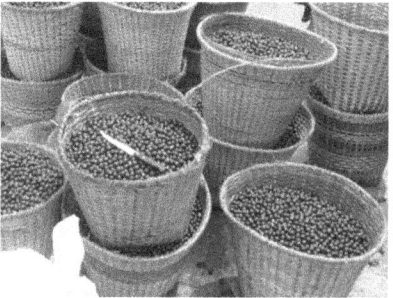

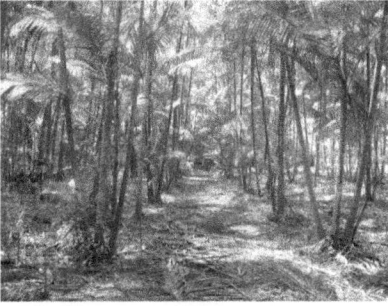

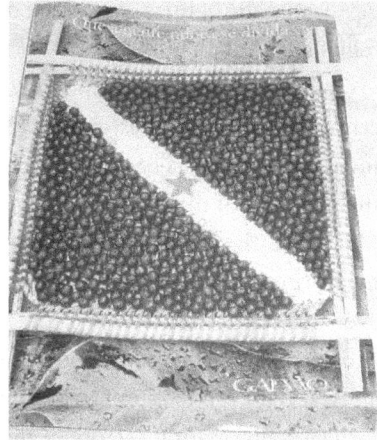

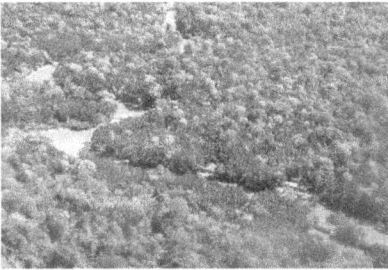

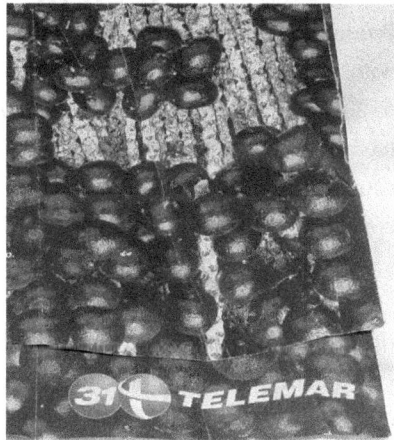

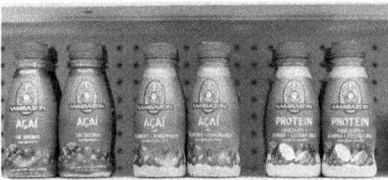

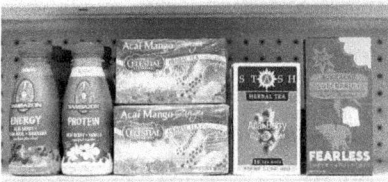

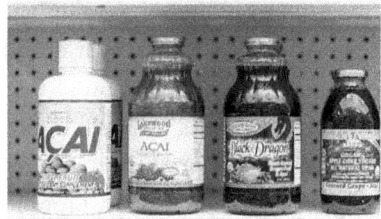

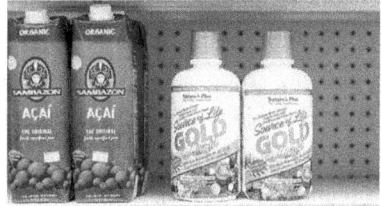

Figure 9.1a Symbolic values and narratives associated with the açaí palm and fruit.

permeated the politics of regional development, discourses of sustainability, and regional social identity.

Today, it is virtually impossible to discuss development and conservation, economic opportunities, and inequalities in the Brazilian Amazon without invoking açaí. It has become the most important regional crop and a symbol of the potential of the region's biodiversity to engender regional development (see McDonell, this volume, on the construction of development potential), slowly measuring up to soy and cattle; it is today foundational to the economy of an ever-increasing number of municipalities, small-scale farming families, and urban entrepreneurs throughout the region.

Açaí fruit production has become one of the largest and most economically inclusive agricultural sectors of the Brazilian Amazon. Just on the production side, it involves over 110,000 production units, 90 percent considered family production units.[4] Costa estimated that the growth rate of employment associated with the regional açaí pulp economy was over 12 percent from the mid-1990s to 2011, representing around 125,000 people per year (2016). Income from açaí has afforded sharecroppers and small-scale producers more security, local niche economies to emerge, and an alternative to the dilemma of deforestation versus conservation in the region. Its centrality in regional life has reified its position as a symbol of local and regional pride and a marker of identity.

I have been working with and documenting the story of açaí producers and the social life of açaí palm and fruit since the late 1980s. My concern has been to understand the implications of a rapidly expanding economy for local producers and landscapes, for local consumers who depend on it as a food source, and for regional economic development.[5] In what ways does an expanding economy create opportunities for value aggregation that benefits producers and the larger population? Although the açaí economy represents a story of economic inclusion, today, the region at the center of açaí production continues to fall behind other areas of Brazil in most indicators of human development. Most small-scale açaí producers still depend on government aid and cash transfer programs (Brondizio 2011; Brondizio et al. 2013).

In what follows, I present a brief reflection on the phases of expansion of the açaí fruit economy from a regional staple to a global craze, a process marked by a growing complexity of agents, market chains, technologies, and narratives of açaí's multiple values. First, I examine how local producers, who have engendered açaí's agroforestry intensification, have been underplayed as agents behind açaí's economic expansion. Second, I examine the process of meaning-making and

Adding value through the commodity chain
1 hectare equivalent of açaí fruit

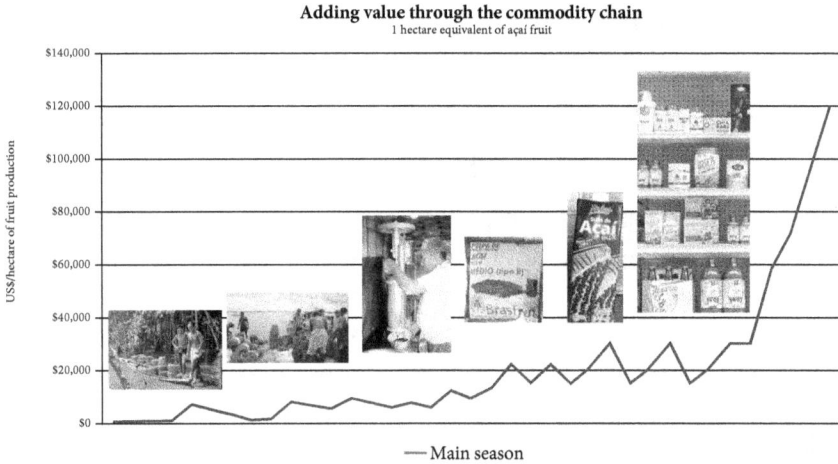

— Main season

Figure 9.1b Value aggregation of the pulp produced in 1 hectare of açaí fruit.

value creation associated with the transformation of açaí for an expanding consumption basis and, in turn, its impact on local low-income consumers. These two processes, the framing of açaí production and the creation of symbolic and economic values, are closely interconnected and have had direct implication for the distribution of benefits of this expanding economy. On the one hand, açaí shows both the potential of local agroforestry knowledge and small-scale production to respond to market opportunities, and, on the other hand, the persistent colonial position of the Amazon within global market chains, that is, exporting raw material that aggregate value proportionally to their distance from the region, arresting the potential benefits of an expanding market for local populations and municipalities (Figure 9.1b).

In examining these interactions, I discuss how açaí, as a commodity and as a story, is endowed with interpretive flexibility, that is, allowing for the development and appropriation of multiple narratives about its production, nutritional properties, symbolic meanings, and role in economic development. From its role as low-income staple food to its growth as an inclusive and agroforestry-based production system to its nutritional and health claims as a superfood, the expansion of açaí as a material commodity cannot be separated from its transformation as a symbolic good,[6] and both are intertwined with the social-economic history of its region of origin. I conclude with a brief reflection on the implication of the açaí globalization story for small-scale producers and for the Amazon.

Framing Agroforestry as Extractivism[7]

Esther Boserup once said: "Any classification of the systems of land use with respect to the degree of intensity is necessarily arbitrary to some extent" (1965, 15). This could not be truer than in the açaí fruit production system.

The açaí palm has been managed along the eastern Amazonian floodplains for centuries, as captured in archeological records and in eighteenth- and nineteenth-century travel accounts and natural history accounts. The current regional economy of açaí and the expansion of açaí fruit production started in the late 1970s and early 1980s, largely as a response to the growing demand for açaí fruit in urban centers of the region. Replacing a declining açaí heart-of-palm economy, açaí fruit had already become a major food production phenomenon in the Amazon estuary-delta region before it had taken off in the mid-1990s as a production system supplying national and international markets. This expansion was based on a combination of the intensification of local agroforestry systems and the progressive expansion of floodplain forest management, both of which are based on local techniques (including forest thinning, selective cutting, pruning, planting, vertical and horizontal intercropping, variety selection, and annual maintenance). In essence, these techniques transform the açaí palm (the plant is a clump with multiple stems) into the dominant production unit in an area, forming diverse configurations of açaí agroforestry, or, as locally called, *açaízais* (Brondizio 2008). These techniques were progressively enhanced and disseminated based on the exchange of experiences among farmers, but also with support from studies of riverside agroforestry (e.g., Anderson et al. 1985 and many others) and the participation of research and extension institutions and NGOs.

The impact of agroforestry and forest management techniques on the production of açaí fruit is tremendous. Açaí palm management is undertaken at the plant (clump and stems) and forest levels, which makes this agricultural transformation not easily recognized by outsiders and potentially invisible or disregarded if one takes a dichotomic view of between forest and agriculture. For instance, in an unmanaged floodplain forest, the "importance value" of açaí palm (a combination of frequency, density, and dominance of a given species in relation to others) lies between 18 percent and 30 percent. As açaí farmers manage and plant these areas, the importance value of açaí palm rises to 70 percent and in some cases more. Different than monocropping, most small-scale producers along the floodplains tend to maintain a diversity of other useful species or crops, precisely because açaí fruit production depends on pollinators that depend on other species to reproduce (Campbell et al. 2018). The number of açaí clumps and stems per hectare increases five- to ten-fold from unmanaged to intensively managed agroforestry. Along the floodplains, farmers maintain interspersed areas of intermediate to highly intensive areas where the density of the production unit can average from 500 clumps/2,000 stems per hectare to over 1,200 clumps/3,000 stems per hectare, respectively. The level of density of the latter, that is, an intensively managed açaí agroforestry, is equivalent to that recommended for monocultural açaí in upland areas, usually requiring irrigation. The productivity harnessed in these systems is equally impressive, increasing from 1–2 tons/ha in unmanaged forests to 4–6 tons/ha in sites of intermediate intensity to 8–12 tons/ha in intensively managed sites, the latter equivalent or superior to açaí monocropping plantations (Brondizio 2008). Productivity varies widely in these sites because of variation in cycles of management, the density of other species and other environmental factors. In sum, it has been through the knowledge and hands of riverine farmers that açaí production has increased from an estimated 25,000 tons in the early 1970s to about 50,000 tons in 1980, 137,000 tons in 1986, and 443,000 tons in 2018 (IBGE 2018a, 2018b).[8]

Ironically, as the açaí economy and production base expanded, small-scale riverine açaí fruit production became framed and narrated as a system of extractivism and, as a consequence, its producers as passive extractivists.[9] The development of this narrative has been based on transposing a historical social category, the extractivist, to the açaí agroforestry production system, regardless of its agronomic qualities. "Extractivism" as a regional economic category is intrinsically associated with social categories such as rubber-tappers, caboclos, and ribeirinhos, encoding their positions at the base of the regional social hierarchy. The social category of extractivist associated with riverine residents was consolidated during the rubber economy in the nineteenth and early twentieth centuries, but it has been re-signified in various ways since the 1980s. On the one hand, the extractivist identity has become the banner of social movements for land rights, as in the case of rubber-tappers (Schmink 2011) and others; on the other hand, the term has served as a general designation for several rural and forest economies, as in the case of açaí. Consolidated in the social hierarchy of the region, the extractivist social category not only prevailed but has been reinforced throughout the economic expansion of açaí.

The irony is that while the region observed a phenomenal expansion of açaí fruit production through the hands of small-scale riverine farmers, its image as a product of native forests harvested by local extractors has been reinforced in academic, policy, and popular narratives. In a telling representation of this reality, a news article (among many examples) describing how a new company is teaching local producers about how to manage and cultivate açaí (i.e., repackaging local management knowledge), the following portrayal emerges:

> Integrated with nature, they know the hour and direction of tides and the dangers of the forest, such as confronting a jaguar during harvesting, but they do not know agricultural techniques that increase açaí production, a palm typical of the Amazon region ... before that, the producer would only see the açaí tree during harvesting.
>
> (Suplemento Agrofolha, Folha de São Paulo, 2003)

Paradoxically, an economy that is born from local knowledge and practices is repositioned as a contribution from new agents who can rationalize and "agronomize" the same practices of the local productive system.

Agronomically and aesthetically, açaí agroforestry defies the perception of clean and homogeneous, domesticated land that has characterized the agrarian history of Brazil since the late sixteenth century. An açaí agroforest can be seen as a messy, complex ecosystem or the most agronomically sophisticated intercropping system. It is beautiful, it is untidy, it is organized, it is chaotic depending on the eyes of the beholder. In Brazil, the social and legal recognition of productive land and private property have been historically based on the cultural concept of land "cleanness." Keeping the land "clean" from forests or secondary vegetation (or savanna) is a way of expressing a farmer's work ethic and technical ability and the social value of property. A production system such as the açaí agroforestry hardly fits the rigid dichotomy between forest and agriculture, productive and unproductive.

There are also historical reasons for such invisibility. For much of the region's colonial history, the majority of riverine families were sharecroppers, indentured servants, or had, at best, customary land rights, as many still do today.[10] Demonstrating "land improvement" based on deforestation and planting of annual crops increases the ability of sharecropper tenants to claim land rights, thus representing a threat to absent landowners. In such a context, the way riverine farmers have managed agroforestry systems, such as açaí, can be seen as a form of everyday resistance. Nurturing forests into "invisible" production systems (built upon local forest species, ethnobotanical knowledge, and low-cost technology) minimized the risk of expulsion by absentee landowners. In this sense, the view of the açaí agroforestry as an extractivist economy also reflects the historical stereotype associated with riverine residents (and extractivism) as lazy ("only see the açaí tree during harvesting") and ignorant ("they do not know agricultural techniques that increase açaí production"), and commonly invoked as a "social pathology" impeding regional development (Nugent 1993). While riverine açaí producers have gained a more positive image, it is still inherently attached to the image of extractivism, an image further reinforced with the expansion of monocultural açaí in upland areas.

From Local to Global Consumption: Meaning-Making, Transformation, and Value Aggregation

The transformation of açaí fruit from a local unsweetened main dish to a multitude of sweetened and blended food items that appeal to a wide range of urban consumers was marked by a shift not only in form, taste, and composition but also in terms of the symbolic value it carries for different groups of people. In this sense, the expansion of the açaí economy benefited from açaí's interpretative flexibility, that is, a fruit that encodes multiple material and symbolic meanings and narrative possibilities: a blessed food staple, a marker of regional identity, a healthy and youthful energy drink, a connection to indigenous Amazonia, a development solution for the Amazon, a mystical exotic forest product, a new type of agriculture, a fruit blessed with superlative biochemical and nutritional properties. The coevolution of açaí's material transformations and meanings underlies its expansion, from local to global spheres, from a staple to a fashion food to a superfood and a symbol of sustainability.

In the eastern Amazon, açaí juice is consumed fresh and daily as part of a meal. In the region, the fresh pulp of açaí is referred to as *vinho do açaí* (literally translated, açaí wine) (Siqueira and Brondizio 2012). It is a purplish liquid of varying thickness depending on the amount of water dilution. In general, mixed generously with manioc flour, it is eaten with a spoon rather than drunk. Fresh açaí is an acquired taste; it is "roughly creamy, metallic, and slightly oily" (Rogez 2000), and it has a mild earth-like taste. In addition to its high energetic value, açaí pulp is rich in fibers, protein, lipids, vitamins such as A, C, E, and B1, minerals such as calcium and potassium, and fiber. Indeed, açaí pulp is recognized to have superlative antioxidant properties. Three main kinds of açaí wine are sold fresh daily in the thousands of small processing stalls throughout urban areas of the region: thick/special, medium, thin/popular. The thickness of açaí (besides origin, ripeness, and overall quality) defines its price to local consumers, as discussed below (see Figure 9.3).

As açaí consumption and uses expanded nationally and globally, it has become associated less with its material qualities, and often irrespective of that, than for what it came to represent to different groups of people. Although one can find high-quality frozen açaí pulp in many parts of the world, many products claiming and advertising açaí barely have any trace of it; they gain economic value by fetishizing açaí's name, images, and stories. Conversely, besides its availability, the value of açaí as a local staple food is based on its material qualities: ripeness, freshness, fatness, and thickness. As açaí pulp is transformed into a multitude of products for new consumers—beverages, snacks, sweets, concentrates, powder, ice creams, vitamins, cosmetics, remedies, and so forth—the material qualities of açaí fruit pulp that are valued locally are replaced by a semiotic combination of signs, images, and narratives associated with its name and nutritional virtues, indigeneity and exoticness, and connections to sustainability.

Likewise, many companies associating their name with the sustainability of açaí production are not directly involved with local producers, communities, or sustainability practices. Independently associating a company's supply chain to açaí production, or with forest extractivism, connects it to a productive and inclusive agroforest-based economy, largely organic and not linked to deforestation. And there lies açaí's power as a symbolic good. Açaí has enough interpretive flexibility to be appropriated and mobilized as a boundary object by and between producers, market actors, researchers, politicians, industries, media, social movements, the regional population, and groups of consumers in different parts of the world (Figures 9.1a and 9.2).

Changing Meanings and Narratives along Phases of Expansion, Transformation, and Consumption

The meanings and narratives of açaí have coevolved with the phases of expansion of its production, industrial, and consumption basis, which, for analytical purposes, can be organized in four overlapping periods (Figure 9.2). Multiple stories and narratives about açaí as a superfood have evolved along the process and have taken on a life of their own. As an "indigenous staple," açaí was part of the diet of indigenous populations occupying large areas of the estuary-delta region prior to and post-European arrival and colonial expansion. Indigenous populations throughout the Amazon consume açaí fruit today. As a "riverine

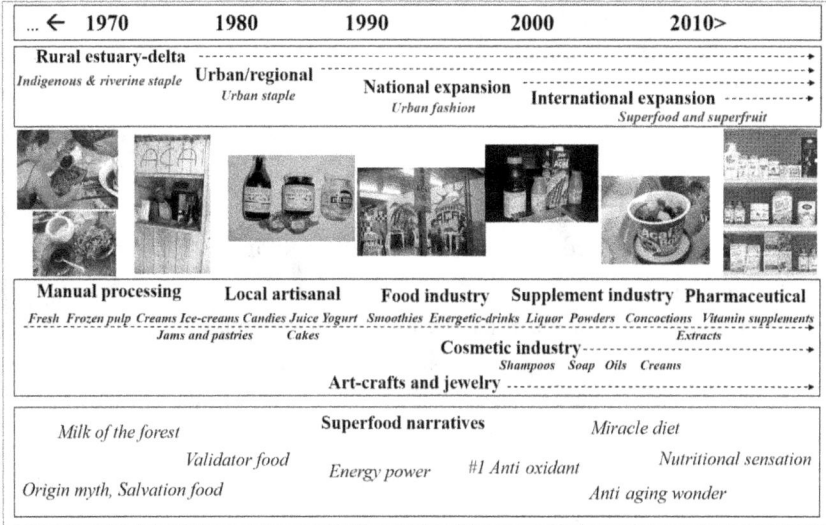

Figure 9.2 Phases of expansion in transformation and consumption of açaí fruit, from a regional staple to a national favorite to an international craze.

rural staple," the consumption of açaí fruit dates back to the seventeenth century, expanding during the period of directorate policies (mid-eighteenth century) and the rubber economic boom (mid-nineteenth century). During the last fifty years, açaí consumption continued to grow in importance among riverine families and communities, the main producers of açaí, throughout the estuary-delta region.

The importance of açaí as a "regional urban staple" led to its first phase of large-scale expansion, as demand for açaí increased rapidly as a low-cost staple food in regional urban centers. This process took place during the 1970s and 1980s and was associated with urban population growth, as rural migrants brought their food culture, taste preference, familiarity, and the need for accessible food items, particularly, but not only, to state capitals such as Belém and Macapá. Locals talk with emotion about the "magical flavor" of açaí and its importance in everyone's diet, from babies to the elderly. An older generation of local producers talk about this period as the onset of the "açaí boom," the *açaização*, of the Amazon estuary-delta region (Hiraoka 1994). Pulp extraction technology had a direct influence on the expansion of açaí as an urban staple. The development and dissemination of electric machines in the late 1960s used to pulp açaí replaced the traditional *amassadeiras de açaí* (women who crush the fruit by hand), allowing the provisioning of expanding demand (Mourão 1999). Estimates of annual per capita consumption of fresh açaí in its main area of production range from 15 to 60 liters/person, with the highest amount among families with the lowest income (Bezerra et al. 2016; Rogez 2000). As noted by Rogez (2000), açaí consumption in the region is twice that of milk. Açaí also has a historical place in celebrated regional desserts, particularly among the regional elite, including ice cream and popsicles, creams, and cakes. In fact, açaí was appreciated as ice cream when the first iceboxes were introduced to the state capital Belém around the beginning of the twentieth century.

After 1990, along with the popularization of other Amazonian fruits outside the region, açaí fruit consumption expanded to other parts of Brazil into what I have called the beginning of its consumption as a "fashion food"; international consumption followed rapidly (Brondizio 2004, 2008). During the first phase of national and international expansion, industrial processing was minimum, focusing on the production and export of frozen pulp, usually with the addition of guarana syrup, making it sweeter. Açaí fruit and pulp spoil quickly, the former molding and decaying and the latter coagulating. For this reason, frozen açaí pulp started to be exported to other regions with the addition of guarana syrup to disguise its original unsweetened taste, which becomes very pronounced with coagulation. Initially exported mainly in the form of frozen pulp packages, açaí fruit was served first as smoothies (*suco de açaí*) or in bowls (*açaí na tijela*) in food huts serving surfers on popular beaches in Rio de Janeiro (e.g., Ipanema, Barra, Leblon, and Copacabana) and in gyms, boosted by the promotion of açaí by the Gracie family, who are originally from Belém and considered founders of Brazilian Jiujitsu.

Açaí bowls are mixed and decorated with fruits, granola, powdered milk, condensed milk, and a creative array of additives, forms of consumption never imagined or considered taboo in its area of origin. Soon, the popularity of açaí juice spread to gym lounges, shopping centers, and progressively to a wide range of *lanchonetes* (sandwich shops); specialized açaí fruit stores (*açaíterias and açaí bars*) emerged throughout Brazil with menus presenting dozens of variations of mixed açaí pulp. From surf shops and gyms, açaí consumption entered into Brazilian soap operas and TV shows. By the late 1990s, açaí had become a recognized icon for health- and body-minded teenagers and adults alike in urban areas throughout the country. In parallel, açaí gained association with environmental sustainability and social inclusion.

As açaí gained an ever-growing consumption basis, a phase of "industrialization" emerged already in the 1990s, initially in the food industry and progressively into cosmetics and pharmaceutical products, each targeting different groups of consumers, from the youth to elders. During this period, new small-scale artesian shops also emerged in the Amazon producing an array of jewelry and art-crafts, as well as local medicines (e.g., cough syrup, energy potions), beauty products (e.g., shampoo, conditioner, soaps), and new food and drink items mixed with chocolate, açaí jams, candies, and liquors. Recently, the pit of açaí, an abundant by-product mostly used as fertilizer or burned as fuel, has been roasted and ground to produce what is being called "açaí coffee."[11] New technology, such as dry freezing, for pulping and storing açaí pulp became central to the expansion of industrialization and export of açaí, eliminating the need for adding guarana syrup and allowing the storage of large stocks for export. The juice, yogurt, and ice-cream industries were among the first to jump in with a variety of flavor combinations. Pasteurized container versions of açaí juice sweetened with guarana syrup and Gatorade-like beverages were launched by the hundreds into the market. Large food corporations, such as McDonald's, started to serve açaí as part of their menus in Brazil. The industries for these products range in location but are mainly in southeast and southern Brazil or internationally, in the United States but later expanded to Europe and Japan. Today, these products are available in supermarkets throughout Brazil and in most large cities around the globe, and specialized açaí bars are currently expanding, particularly in the United States.

In the early 2000s, as açaí was becoming known as a nutritive energetic beverage in Brazil, the United States, and beyond, new narratives about its pharmaceutical qualities emerged along with increasing biochemical research and the development of a multitude of health products. By 2004, mega-celebrity Oprah Winfrey endorsed açaí as the world's number one superfood. The appropriation and remaking of narratives associated with açaí's superpowers took a life on its own. Hundreds of food products, concentrates and supplements, and cosmetics emerged promoting açaí miracle cures and diet, almost always comparing its nutritional and biochemical properties to other superfoods.

Many of these products only slightly remind one of açaí fruit's taste as consumed in its place of origin. Their narratives focus on promoting açaí's energetic and pharmaceutical values and its connections to multiple causes associated with the Amazon. Claims about the product focus on statements such as "the power of the Amazon," "Amazon's milk," "shamans' power," "#1 superfood," among others. However, more so than in the national market, açaí's international expansion gained a stronger emphasis on the environmental and developmental advantages of açaí fruit production as sustainable; it also comes to symbolize fair trade and other forms of supporting local communities. Through the consumption of açaí, the consumer is put in direct touch with the symbolic power of Amazonian nature, indigenous wisdom, and a socioenvironmental cause.

Value Aggregation away from the Region and the Impact of Inflation on Low-Income Consumers

While most of regional açaí production is consumed in the Amazon region, export continues to increase as the consumption for açaí pulp continues to grow nationally and internationally and new industrial uses emerge. A combination of a solid regional market and the fast expansion of external markets and transformation industries underlies the increasingly complex socioeconomic structure now in place in the açaí economy, intertwined with the equally complex system of land and resource ownership in the Amazon. For producers, capturing the economic benefits from an expanding market has been strongly based on one's land tenure condition (particularly for sharecroppers), level of access to infrastructure (particularly transportation), and type of price agreement with buyers (e.g., daily or seasonal contracts). Because açaí fruit spoils within three days, dependence on middlemen and transportation cost can severely affect profitability. The emergence of an export sector and transformation industries has created periods of high inflation of the local value of açaí, directly affecting local consumers. On the other hand, most fruit-producing municipalities do not have fruit processing industries and as such have minimal participation in value aggregation. As Figure 9.1b illustrates, the value of açaí fruit and pulp (i.e., from the producer to the market to urban vendors to frozen pulp for export) may increase by fiftyfold after leaving the farmers' hand and many-fold higher once it is converted into industrial products.

The national and international expansion of the açaí fruit economy had a direct impact on local consumption, particularly among low-income urban and rural residents. After 2000, the inflation of the price of fresh açaí hit hard both local processors and consumers. Between 2006 and 2007, as part of ethnographic research among açaí processors and consumers, we were able to record daily prices for one açaí fruit basket (15 kg) and one liter of fresh açaí (thick/special, medium, thin/popular) in four açaí stalls in the capital and interior of the state of Pará. The wealth generated by the açaí export economy was affecting the very core of local diet and food culture, a topic widely discussed in local newspapers and radio shows. Dilution and adulteration of açaí pulp became commonplace, particularly during the off-season when the price of açaí baskets can reach very high prices (Figure 9.3).

To compensate for fruit price increases, local processors started diluting the pulp of açaí thin/popular (and to some extent medium) to the extreme: "it is pure tinted water" as I heard many times from both processors and consumers. As price continued to increase, processors selling açaí in low-income areas (the

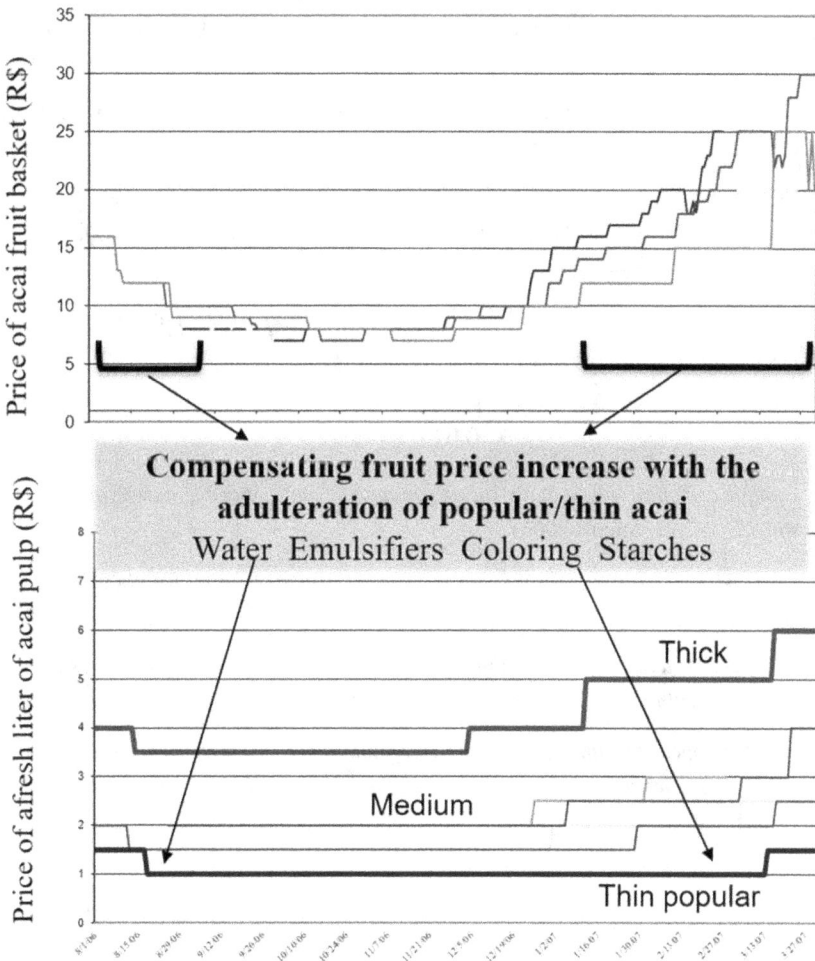

Figure 9.3 Data from four açaí processors, 2006–7, Ponta de Pedras and Belém, Pará State.

majority) started to add food dyes, manioc flour, and corn starch, and even ice-cream emulsifiers as thickeners; to keep consumers coming they had to keep prices as low as possible throughout the year. A series of vignettes collected during fieldwork is illustrative of these dynamics:

Processors/vendors

To make any profit I had to make 30 liters of açaí from this single basket; and people still buy it! Some people need it, they cannot live without it. I use corn starch, beets, and ice cream emulsifier when I need to. (Interior, August 2006)

The Marajoara has to drink açaí even if it is no more than dirt water; one just wants to make sure it is part of a meal. (Interior, July 2008)

Here in the periphery, price came close to R$4 when a basket was selling for R$40, but I could not sell it any higher because people here just cannot pay for it. (Belem, July 2008)

This year was terrible, the price of a basket reached R$45, so I had to sell "water." (Belem, July 2007)

Consumers

I found a blob of wheat flour inside my açaí … no wonder it makes me feel stuffed. (Belem, August 2006)

It is pure water, but people buy it because otherwise they do not feel they had a good lunch. (Interior, July 2007)

The açaí is so adulterated that it makes me feel bloated, with heart-burn, but still, I can't live without it. (Interior, July 2007)

I just stopped consuming it when I cannot afford a better açaí (thicker), but my dad must have it every day, so here I am to buy his açaí. (Belem, August 2006)

In spite of the significant increase in açaí fruit production in the region, its international market continues to expand, and inflation continues to be a concern for Amazonian consumers.

Concluding Thoughts

On many grounds, the açaí story is a tale of success. Açaí fruit has never been as important to the regional economy as today, and not surprisingly, throughout the region açaí fruit is considered a blessing, a superfruit, one that provides both a beloved food source and an unrivaled source of income. Yet, while local producers and the region have benefited greatly from the economy they have created, progressively the largest share of the booming açaí market—the value aggregation through the material and symbolic transformation of the fruit—is captured elsewhere. The lack of transformation industries that aggregate value to açaí in the region has limited the ability of municipalities, mostly struggling and insolvent, to capture tax benefits from industrial transformation and jobs for the local youth (Brondizio 2011). The commercialization of açaí fruit, as with other resource economies in the Amazon, runs from the hands of producers to family-middleman-broker networks to local consumers and corporations, thus bypassing the formal economy of municipalities. Not surprisingly, the scale of the açaí fruit economy is many times that of the budget and revenues of the municipalities where it is produced. As a story relevant to many other crops and regions, multimillion-dollar local açaí economies co-exist with some of the most insolvent and poor municipal realities.

Returning to the main title above, the açaí story encapsulates the possibilities and predicaments associated with the globalization of local food systems and invites us to reflect on the position of small-scale farmers within larger market chains. As in other cases in this volume, such as that of quinoa, the açaí story shows that the expansion of local agricultural economies goes through quickly evolving phases, marked by changes in agents' markets, narratives, technologies, regulations, and institutions, all of which have implications for shifting economic opportunities (Brondizio 2004, 2008). As new entrepreneurs enter the supply chain, small-scale producers are both romanticized and dismissed in their ability to respond to market demands. As in the case of açaí, the unfavorable position of riverine small-scale farmers in the region has been reasserted by new agents and in narratives reproducing historical-cultural and economic stereotypes. In this process, local knowledge has been repackaged and reintroduced as new agents gain positions in a profitable production system. As production areas expand and supply balances demand, profit and surplus shift progressively to other sectors and agents, such as processing, controlling product stocks and export, and the transformation industries and distributors. The lack of policy incentives and infrastructure supporting a larger participation of the regional population in processing, transformation, and commercialization of this valuable superfruit arrests benefits to the region as a whole. Today, the açaí story puts the Amazon at a crossroads: to pursue an inclusive and transformative economy based on its biodiversity and local knowledge, adding value to its resources to benefit the regional population, or to maintain its colonial position and destructive land use.

Many hopeful signs are also emerging. Some industries are starting to be located in the region, while others are seeking to engage directly with local producers. Throughout the interior of the region, small-scale producers and rural communities are creating new micro-scale pulp industries, forming local cooperatives and collective financing mechanisms. New programs, such as the inclusion of fresh açaí in public schools, have created opportunities for producers to process and sell açaí directly at a higher price. However, significant constraints remain in terms of agricultural credit, support for sanitary compliance, processing and storage facilities, transportation, and support for commercialization. For Amazonian small-scale farmers, challenges are always ahead of opportunities.

Currently, the Brazilian government is aggressively expanding commodity production and promoting deforestation as a pathway to "development" of the Amazon, taking away the rights of and disregarding the contributions of indigenous peoples and local populations to the region. In this context, the açaí story offers powerful counterfactual evidence, an alternative narrative, and a reflexive mirror of the possibilities and predicaments of the region. Lessons learned from the açaí story could give hope of a more inclusive and sustainable future for the Amazon.

Acknowledgments

I appreciate the contribution of numerous producers and agents involved with the açaí economy, Andrea D. Siqueira and multiple collaborators with whom I have worked in the region since the late 1980s; Emma McDonell and Richard Wilk for their invitation and helpful comments on the manuscript. Over the years, this work has received support from multiple agencies, most recently from the National Science Foundation (Grant #072972) in support of the project *Agents: Amazonian Governance to Enable Transformations to Sustainability*, which also has support from FAPESP (Brazil), NW0 (The Netherlands), Vetenskapsradet (Sweden), all of which are part of the Transformation to Sustainability research program organized by NORFACE and the Belmont Forum. This chapter is also part of the project *Emerging Areas of Research—Sustainable Food System Sciences (SFSS)*. I am also thankful for the support of my department and Indiana University.

Notes

1 The myth of origin of açaí portrays a drama of famine, infanticide, tears, and the miracle salvation provided by a superfood. A short version goes as: "In the place known today as Belém (the capital of the state of Pará in the Brazilian Amazon), once upon a time there was a large Indian group facing a scarcity of food. In order to control population growth, the chief decided that every newborn child would have to be sacrificed. Shortly after this order was given, the chief's own daughter, Iaçá, gave birth to a beautiful girl. She too was soon sacrificed. Iaçá was very sad and desperate, and every night she cried. One full moon night, she listened to a baby cry and when she got out of her hamlet, she saw her daughter close to a palm tree. Full of hope and happiness, Iaçá ran to hug her daughter. As soon as she did it, the girl disappeared mysteriously. The next morning the other villagers found Iaçá dead and hugging the palm tree. In her face they could still see her happiness and her black eyes stared at a palm that was full of little purple-black fruits. The chief ordered the fruits harvested and made a tasty juice with them. This fruit provided enough food for everyone, and soon the chief suspended his order and babies were allowed to live. The chief named the fruit palm açaí in honor of his daughter Iaçá, the fruit that cries."

2 Açaí from the Tupi language (also *Yasa"y(i)*, *Içá-çaí*, *Assai*) meaning crying fruit, fruit with water, or palm of the water. Scientific name: *Euterpe oleracea Mart,* from the Greek *Euterpe*, meaning grace or pleasure. A multistem palm, it produces fruit bunches of small purple-black drupes. It occurs naturally in the Amazon estuary-delta and surrounding regions, where it is often referred to as the tree of life.

3 Many uses of the palm are losing importance as locals have more access to plastic and other materials.

4 66,296 production units are considered "extractivist" (or 60 percent of total units) of which 92 percent are considered family units, and 47,855 production units are considered agricultural, of which 86 percent are considered family production units (IBGE 2017, 2018a, 2018b).

5 In this text, I speak particularly about the region at the center of açaí fruit production in the Amazon, the estuary-delta region and surroundings, which includes around fifty municipalities in two Brazilian states, Pará and Amapá. Today,

açaí fruit is produced throughout the Amazon region, but the estuary-delta region remains the most important center of production. The estuary-delta region as referred here is broadly equivalent to what Costa (2016) refers to as the *Grão Pará* region.

6   This is a loose analogy to Bourdieu's analysis of cultural production (1971), which I still find useful.

7   This section overlaps partially with an article written in Portuguese for the Brazilian report on indigenous and traditional local communities: "Contributions for Biodiversity, Threats, and Public Policies," edited by Manuela Carneiro da Cunha, Sônia B. M. Santos, and Cristina Adams (n.d.).

8   Even though impressive, I consider these figures to be underestimated. Rogez (2000), for instance, estimated production to be closer to 500,000 tons by the year 2000. Since the 1990s, and particularly after 2000, açaí production expanded to the Amazon as a whole. Currently, it is expanding to other parts of Brazil and other countries. This expansion included the intensification of açaí agroforestry in the floodplains and planting of açaí in upland areas, both in small-scale agroforestry systems and in large-scale monocultural plantations, using new varieties of upland/dry soil açaí developed by the Brazilian agropastoral research agency EMBRAPA. This expansion has allowed the inclusion of a large number of small-scale farmers previously depending on manioc shifting cultivation, off-farm employment, and in some cases cattle ranching. The largest expansion taking place currently, however, is that of large-scale plantations, in many cases replacing pastures or secondary forests. Since 2015, IBGE has included planted açaí areas in its assessment, but estimates vary significantly among reports; for instance for the North region, it ranges from 273 million (IBGE 2017) to 1.5 million tons (IBGE 2018a).

9   In the mid-1990s, we argued that açaí production is a system of "forest farming" by "forest farmers" (Brondizio and Siqueira 1997).

10   Since the 1990s, there has been significant improvement in land titling throughout the region. The agricultural census indicates that today most açaí producers are considered "landowners."

11   To my knowledge, this product was developed by a women's association, AMABELA, in the Belterra Municipality in the lower Amazon and Tapajos river region.

10

Amaranth's "Rediscovery" in Mexico: A Path Toward Decolonization of Food?

Florence Bétrisey and Valérie Boisvert

In the early 2010s, online media began to hail a "new and highly nutritious crop" as a superfood (Bruce 2014). Some articles described amaranth as "the next quinoa" and projected that it was about to "join quinoa, chia seeds and goji berries in the pantheon of ancient 'superfoods' enjoying a much-deserved resurgence" (Maisto 2011). According to enthusiastic and widely quoted reports from journalists, the ancient crop would make a comeback in its native Mexico (Howard 2013), thanks to the pioneering initiatives of American volunteers in support of local NGOs (Matsumoto 2017; Slow Food 2007). International NGOs, development organizations, and Mexican and international media outlets alike gave glowing accounts of the role that amaranth would play in the fight against malnutrition and obesity along with the revival of Aztec culinary traditions lost during colonization. This constellation of institutional actors has gradually crafted and deployed a narrative about amaranth over the last decade, describing what it will achieve once widely grown and consumed, and summoning desirable futures with political, material, and ontological implications in the present. This recent "rediscovery" deserves all the more attention as it reflects a radical and to a large extent unstated shift in the representation of amaranth.

Grain amaranths are pseudo-cereals belonging to the genus *Amaranthus L.* of the family *Amaranthaceae*, which encompasses about seventy species (Mapes Sanchez and Basurto Peña 2016).[1] Wherever amaranth is grown, it seems to be associated with "non- or second-class citizens," such as slaves and black communities in Jamaica and economic migrants in Malaysia (De Shield 2015, 6). Some of the species are native to the Americas, where amaranth was a significant crop for many pre-Columbian societies (Das 2012). Like quinoa in the Andes (see McDonell, this volume), amaranth is pejoratively considered as an *comida de indios* in contemporary Mexico (Velasco Lozano 2017) and has long been marginalized under neocolonial mentalities. The reimagining of amaranth as a "superfood" raises a number of critical questions about the politics of discovery narratives and their role in culinary revalorization projects. Beyond the seemingly simple story line, what does the rediscovery of amaranth in Mexico stand for? What exactly is being rediscovered, by whom, and for whom? What are the stakes? Drawing on discourse analysis (Hajer 2006) and the sociology of expectations (Borup et al. 2006; Joly 2013), this chapter aims to unpack the discourse surrounding amaranth's rediscovery in Mexico. We offer a critical examination of its possible contribution to a process of decolonization of food and diet, in the sense of Peña et al. (2017).

Hajer's argumentative discourse analysis aims at highlighting how discourses "shape one's view of the world and reality" (Hajer and Versteeg 2005, 176) and influence laws and institution building. The notion of *framing*, understood as a discursive process whereby political actors "aim to create necessities for (specific) policy intervention" through argumentation (Leipold and Winkel 2016, 36), is used to unpack the embeddedness of discourse in practices and politics (Hajer and Versteeg 2005). Through framing, actors create *story lines* which are "condensed statement[s] summarizing complex narratives, used by people as 'short hand' in discussions" (Hajer 2006, 69). These story lines both empower some actors and entail discursive *delegitimation* and exclusion of others by, for example, not referring to them (Leipold and Winkel 2016).

The framing of amaranth's rediscovery shares a particular kind of narrative based on promises about the plant and its ability to solve urgent development and health problems. The analysis of promissory narratives developed in the sociology of expectations (Borup et al. 2006; Brown and Michael 2003; Joly 2013) has proven a fruitful approach to the study of techno-scientific innovations, their legitimation, and their dissemination. For instance, Pierre-Benoit Joly (2013) identified a number of stylized facts related to the diffusion of biotechnologies: the formulation of a promise to solve a general and urgent problem (world hunger, environmental crisis), made credible by scientific studies and the personal commitment of scientists, and supported by some success stories that everyone is referring to. Paradoxically, radical opposition to the promise makes it more plausible. The promise gradually becomes an "obligatory passage point" (Akrich et al. 2006), building collective commitment, mutually binding obligations, and agendas for action. Working on cultured meat, Sexton et al. (2019) convincingly showed how "promissory narratives" were effective in promoting new technologies. Taking the notion beyond the field of technology, Foyer et al. (2017) have explored the way promises could also explain the consensus around market-based instruments for biodiversity conservation. We consider the rediscovery of amaranth in Mexico and its consecration as superfood as a promissory narrative to critically examine how it frames the political and moral economy of the plant and singles out some facts and actors while silencing others.

Context

In Mesoamerica, amaranths are estimated to have been domesticated as early as 5000 BC (Das 2012, 274). However, the transition from wild harvest to agriculture occurred gradually and plant geneticists debate the precise moment of domestication (McClung de Tapia 2016). This exemplifies the fact that distinctions between wild and domesticated plants are often blurry and are in any case socially constructed. In Mexico, some farmers would not actively sow amaranths but would welcome wild amaranth plants in or around fields, even watering them and letting them go to seed to ensure their reproduction (Mapes Sanchez and Basurto Peña 2016).

According to anthropologists Esther Katz and Elena Lazos, Mexico has retained more Amerindian traditions related to food than other countries in Latin America (Katz and Lazos 2017, 20). They argue that this might be due to the existence of a "refined court cuisine" (Katz and Lazos 2017, 22) within the Aztec empire that has been partly adopted by Spanish viceroyalty. After independence in 1821, the "invention of national cuisine" appeared as an important "political project for the new nation" (Katz and Lazos 2017, 22). The 1910 Revolution, by "enhancing the glorification of the indigenous roots of the country" (Katz and Lazos 2017, 22), contributed to the valuing of the numerous dishes that belonged to an indigenous heritage. Mexican food has also suffered from "modernization" projects which have translated into industrialization of so-called "traditional" food like tortillas, the development of a fast-food industry (Pilcher 2012), and the further marginalization of indigenous foodways. Lately, the declaration of traditional Mexican cuisine as intangible heritage by UNESCO in 2010 is said to have generated "tremendous enthusiasm among chefs, entrepreneurs, government institutions and communities, eager to promote both Mexican gastronomical traditions and innovations" (Katz and Lazos 2017, 22).

Amaranth figures as one of these indigenous foods increasingly promoted among Mexican consumers. Pre-Aztec indigenous communities in Central America domesticated two species of amaranth (*Amaranthus cruentus* and *Amaranthus hypocondriacus*) (McClung de Tapia 2016) for grain consumption, while they were gathering wild species of amaranth (*A. hybridus*) for their leaves (Katz and Lazos 2017). Under the Aztec regime, grain amaranth was both a staple and a ritual food, used as tribute like maize (Velasco Lozano 2016). Grain amaranth was ground into flour or toasted and mixed with maize and honey to form figurines eaten during ceremonials (Katz and Lazos 2017). The making of such figurines was prohibited by Spaniards but the crop itself was never banned (Velasco Lozano 2016). Amaranth cultivation is then reported to have gradually declined since the seventeenth century, without completely disappearing (Katz and Lazos 2017). Indeed, it is still consumed in the form of *alegrias*, sweet bars made of popped amaranth and honey, which are a popular street food in Mexico today (McClung de Tapia 2016).

Nowadays, "health-conscious people of the urban intellectual middle class" (Katz and Lazos 2017, 28) consume popped amaranth in their breakfast cereals and consider it as a "health food" (Katz and Lazos 2017, 28). According to Rojas-Rivas et al. (2019), amaranth has even become a marker of social distinction. Mexican amaranth is increasingly exported, mostly to the United States (Katz and Lazos 2017). Amaranth from Tulyehualco has recently been declared "intangible cultural heritage of the city of Mexico" (Velasco Lozano 2017). Scholars, however, consider that amaranth "has not regained its place as a staple and strategic crop" (Espitia Rangel 2016, 66) and hypothesize that hidden power relations may explain why amaranth is "escaping the poorest who need [it] more" (Katz and Lazos 2017, 43).

By analyzing the framing of this "rediscovery" of amaranth in media and in national/international organizations' discourse, we aim at better understanding how power relationships and economic interest crystallize to achieve this elite capture of amaranth as a "superfood."

Methods

We collected our corpus of texts by searching Google for the following keywords: *amaranth rediscovery Mexico, amaranth revival Mexico, amaranto redescubrimiento Mexico, amaranto Mexico*. We then selected texts based on our judgment. We ended up with a corpus of twenty-six texts, ranging from

2007 to 2018 and including twelve international media outlets, seven scientific papers (agricultural science, food science [3], biotechnology, health science, anthropology), three Mexican media outlets, and four documents issued by international non- and inter-governmental organizations.

A plant can only be rediscovered if it was first *discovered*, then somehow faded into oblivion before becoming again the focus of attention. Rediscovery narratives involve summoning the past and giving a subjective and political account of initial discovery and oblivion phases. Accordingly, we coded these three episodes of the "rediscovery" story lines and identified for each the objects at stake (what is discovered/forgotten/revived), the narrative characters (heroes, villains, victims), and their motivations. In a second step, we identified different "promises" at work across different framings of the "problems" in Mexico. Finally, we coded the actors in the rediscovery story line, according to the legitimacy and importance attributed or denied to them (farmers, NGOs, commercial actors, scientists).

Rediscovering What?

The term "superfood" does not correspond to any established scientific or legal category (Loyer and Knight 2018). It could be more accurately described as a "marketing term" (Schiemer et al. 2018) and a "discursive device" (Loyer and Knight 2018, 450) designed to invoke superhero representations and suggest extraordinary powers. Consequently, the qualities or "desirable traits" (Cernansky 2015, 146) highlighted as characteristic of superfood are quite variable. They do not result from a mere comprehensive scientific assessment but follow agricultural and nutritional trends, which in turn are influenced by the broader political context (Kimura 2013). The qualities attributed to amaranth thus reflect the valued features and guiding principles that prevail in this context.

We identified a first set of key features described in terms of presence and absence. This includes the fact that amaranth is "gluten free," which has become a major asset (appearing in twenty-three publications), that it contains "vitamins" (appearing in twenty publications), notably "folic acid" (appearing in eleven publications), and important "amino acids" (appearing in eighteen publications). Significantly, nineteen publications cite at least two of these nutritional qualities together. This suggests that amaranth is considered a "superfood," a "super grain," or a "wonder food" (appearing in nine publications) because of that very combination of nutritional qualities. This is consistent with the analysis of McDonell (2015) on quinoa. In the past, malnutrition was defined as a deficiency of specific nutrients (protein or vitamin A), which justified adding them to foods through biofortification, but a nutritional paradigm shift has brought about a change in this regard. The "hidden hunger" discourse points to the lack of nutrient diversity as the major cause of malnutrition. Emphasis is therefore placed on the need for several nutrients (Kimura 2013).

In addition to being a superfood, amaranth is also portrayed as a "super crop" with outstanding agronomic properties, such as the ability to grow easily (appearing in fifteen publications), even in harsh environments. Other qualities include its "adaptability" or agronomic fitness due to its genetic plasticity (appearing in three publications). The "resistance" and "resilience" of amaranth are also mentioned, literally as well as in a broader, metaphorical sense, legitimating the superfood label (appearing in four publications each). As McDonell (2015) has shown for quinoa, it is the combination of the nutritional and agronomic values of amaranth that makes it not only a "miracle food" but also a miracle crop and allows hyperbole. The term "supercrop" appears in three documents.

Amaranth is also presented as culturally entrenched, "ancient" (appearing in eight publications), "traditional" (appearing in five publications), or "indigenous" (appearing in four publications). The history of the plant is inextricably linked to the fate of ancient civilizations, which gives it a mythical dimension. Five publications refer to the Maya, five to the Inca, while four publications allude to "pre-Columbian" indigenous groups. Most of them refer to the Aztec (nineteen publications). Six publications cite amaranth's vernacular name in Nahuatl (*huautli*) and three its name in Quechua. The stories referring to the Aztec mention the use of amaranth in diet, as a tribute, and mostly in religious rituals. More specifically, they refer to the supposed custom of mixing amaranth with sacrificial blood to form figurines, which were then ingested during ceremonies. This narrative style is reminiscent of the storytelling marketing technique (Salmon 2010):

> It was a favorite food of Huitzilopochtli, the hummingbird-visaged God of War who, legend had it, led the Aztecs out of the country's northern wastelands to become lords of central Mexico. Amaranth flowers are bright and sweet; hummingbirds love them. Huitzilopochtli, like all the gods of old Mexico, also loved the taste of human blood. A regular diet of sacrifices sustained him and kept the world from falling into darkness.

(Elbein 2013)

Such narratives conjure up visions of an idealized past, an age of sensational sacrificial bloodshed and sacred violence, both frightening and appealing.

Guthman (this volume) also shows how "a really good story behind it" is key to the success of superfood. When applied to "exotic" (Huwyler 2016) or "ethnic" (Calderon 2017) superfoods, these stories specifically "appeal to exoticism and nativism coupled with claims of superfood status" (Drew et al. 2017, 266), a combination that Loyer and Knight (2018, 450) call the "nutritional primitivism" discourse, understood as "the promotion of ancient or indigenous foodways as a path to health" and based on the "fetishiz[ation] of the (food) culture of ancient or indigenous peoples" (Loyer and Knight 2018, 456). Combined with references to nutrition science, this discourse serves "to doubly verify superfoods' healthfulness" (Loyer and Knight 2018, 456). This endorsement by modern science backed by tradition appears in some of the names used for amaranth such as "the Aztec super crop" or "ancient superfood" (Bruce 2014; Maisto 2011).

The story of the rediscovery of amaranth as superfood thus contributes to a fetishization of ancient civilizations through a reification of cultural qualities. Otherwise, this narrative reduces amaranth to its modern nutritional and agronomic qualities, considering it as a set of useful nutrients (see Spackman, this volume, on extractionist logics) and desirable traits that make it an adaptable panacea. It supports the rediscovery thesis in conveying the notion of an improved traditional crop and paves the way for promoting amaranth cultivation around the world, a project similar to what is being promoted for quinoa (Bazile et al. 2016; see McDonell, this volume). This grand gest of amaranth's rediscovery is organized in three movements—its discovery, oblivion, and rediscovery—which we called the three moments of the rediscovery.

The Three Moments of Rediscovery

The "discovery" of amaranth is poorly described and framed (for instance, the word *discovery* does not appear in the corpus). Among some sources, it can still be equated with the first domestication of the plant and its use in diet and rituals. However, while archaeologists have found traces of cultivation of amaranth dating back to 5000 BC in Mexico (Russell 2015), well before the rise of the Mayan and Aztec empires, references to pre-Aztec/pre-Mayan Mesoamerican groups are almost nonexistent in media discourses. Other sources seem to equate the discovery of amaranth with the colonial encounter and the first written descriptions of the plant and its cultural relevance: "when the Spanish arrived in Mexico they recognized the significance of amaranth to the indigenous population" (Bruce 2014). Overall, the discovery phase (and both its objects and actors) remains unclear and almost unframed.

On the contrary, the oblivion phase is well documented by concordant sources. Amaranth is reported to have "faded into obscurity" (The Lexicon n.d.), to have been "forgotten" (Zins 2016), and to have gone "into the history books" (Eaton 2013), leading to an "almost total disappearance" (Slow Food 2007). The colonial eradication of amaranth is held responsible for this loss. Stories of banning amaranth and tales of amaranth growers whose hands were cut off or who were sentenced to death, and of a "religious purge of amaranth" (Elbein 2013) due to its use in Aztec religious rituals, circulate in the majority of the sources. Although the Spaniards most likely "disdained" amaranth consumption (Katz and Lazos 2017, 20) and prohibited the making of offering figurines, there is no historical evidence of this ban and following punishments (Early 1992; Velasco Lozano 2016). Yet there is no narrative without intrigue and tensions. These additions give dramatic intensity to the story and make it more compelling. Mentions of guilt, blame, and a forbidden crop spice up the narrative. They also allow readers to posit the current rediscovery of amaranth as reparation for historical injustice and to turn it into an ethical undertaking.

Finally, rediscovery per se is described as an ongoing process, produced by a constellation of actors and interests. First, "modern research" (Milner 2015) is portrayed as having played a critical role. Amaranth was already called the "crop of the future" on account of its "outstanding agronomic traits" in the context of agronomic research conducted by the Rodale Research Centre and the US National Academy of Science in the 1970s.[2] Another US National Academy of Science report, entitled "Amaranth: Modern Prospects for an Ancient Crop" and released in 1985, and NASA's introduction of amaranth into astronaut diets have been important milestones in the history of rediscovery. Another major contribution to the rediscovery of amaranth put forward is that of economic actors: "pioneer" (Balderas 2018) micro-businesses began to transform amaranth in the 2000s and Kellogg's began including amaranth in its cereal bars in 2010. Mexican NGOs have been instrumental in the revival of amaranth by "rescuing" (López-Garcia 2008), "re-introducing" (Bruce 2014), "reviving" (Eaton 2013; Matsumoto 2017; Slow Food 2007) the crop, by "pushing an amaranth comeback" (Matsumoto 2017), and by encouraging local farmers to grow amaranth. This is the core of amaranth storytelling. The Mexican rediscovery of amaranth is abundantly reported in the press through interviews with NGO representatives, lively and colorful accounts of workshops and various activities, and pictures. We found that three Mexican NGO projects promoting amaranth were showcased as success stories featured in almost every article on the subject and offered as a practical demonstration of amaranth revival.[3]

This framing of amaranth's rediscovery legitimizes and prescribes courses of actions. The first action, mostly undertaken by NGOs, consists in "convincing" (Howard 2013) and "teaching" (The Lexicon n.d.) farmers to grow and consumers to eat amaranth through workshops, campaigns, and cookbooks. Further measures concern the insertion of amaranth into formal breeding programs, which involves wild crop and farmers' varieties germplasm acquisition and the establishment of *ex-situ* collections to develop new varieties through novel breeding techniques. Finally, the rediscovery narrative supports the completion of amaranth commodification by creating and developing formal markets, following "new market trends" (López-Garcia 2008), and "developing marketable varieties" (Eaton 2013). These courses of actions are in line with the framing of obstacles to the achievement of amaranth promises, namely lack of awareness of the nutritional properties of amaranth, lack of interest from "huge companies" and problems of commercialization, and lack of support from government.

Rediscovery by Whom and for Whom?

Scientists, food companies, and NGOs are imagined to play a pivotal role in the revitalization and modernization of amaranth, which legitimizes and empowers them to carry on their efforts. As previously noted, we found that three Mexican NGOs are repeatedly mentioned as key actors in the rediscovery process. The latter are supported by intergovernmental organizations (e.g., International Fund for Agricultural Development, IFAD) and larger NGOs (e.g., Slowfood International) or private actors (Kellogg's Corporation).

Perhaps more surprisingly, amaranth itself is described as having contributed and collaborated in efforts for its rediscovery, together with farmers who resowed it and with the patronage of NGOs. The crop is personified, depicted as an "orphan" (Kilpatrick 2015), the victim of oblivion and marginalization but is also framed positively as having "survived" (Elbein 2013; Howard 2013; Slow Food 2007), "resurfaced" (Vargas Guadarrama and del Valle Berrocal 2016), or "managed to endure" (Milner 2015) in part by itself. Amaranth is therefore lauded for its "tenacity" (Milner 2015). This can be related to what researchers consider to be the incomplete domestication of amaranth, allowing it to propagate even without human assistance, like its wild relatives.

The part played by farmers in the rediscovery narratives is also decisive since they are ultimately responsible for sowing, planting, managing, and harvesting amaranth. In most accounts, farmers are imagined as the intended beneficiaries of the cultivation and commercialization of amaranth. However, they are discredited in two respects. On the one hand, they are sometimes charged with negligence or nonchalance and stigmatized for having "abandoned" (Eaton 2013) or "forgotten" (Elbein 2013) amaranth for lack of vision. To some extent, they are insidiously made responsible and lectured for changes that have been imposed on them. They are implicitly and somewhat condescendingly blamed for their inability to grasp the importance of their food-crop heritage and to conform to primitivist clichés in this regard. The abandonment of "traditional food" is the source of one of the biggest scourges in Mexico according to the rediscovery narrative framing (Eaton 2013), namely the "obesity epidemic" coupled with malnutrition (Howard 2013). The latter is related to a shift from "traditional-agriculture-based diet" (Kilpatrick 2015) to a heavy reliance on processed food "that lacks nutritious and diverse offerings" (The Lexicon n.d.). On the other hand, farmers are also presented as destitute and purposeless, victims of an "obesogenic and toxic environment" (Kilpatrick 2015), requiring the assistance and guidance of scientists, NGOs, and business actors for farming and cooking amaranth adequately and relearning tradition.

This representation of farmers as victims applies in particular to women. Children and pregnant women are framed as "at particular risk of malnutrition which can be severe and irreversible, perpetuating a cycle of poverty" (Bruce 2014). Women are the main targets of cooking classes and awareness raising on the nutritional and health benefits of amaranth in light of their role in household food management determined by local gendered norms. In addition, the high folic acid content of amaranth makes it particularly suitable for pregnant women to reduce birth defects, which are framed as one of the major health issues in Mexico. This focus on women is quite visible in the pictures illustrating papers and reports. Out of eleven pictures showing only women, four show women in (cooking) workshops, two in food stores, three show women processing or cooking amaranth, and one represents a woman carrying her child. By contrast, men are mostly shown working in the fields. This tends to reinforce social expectations aligning women with reproductive tasks. While some sources promise that growing amaranth will "help impoverished women" (Eaton 2013) or "provide women with livelihoods" (The Lexicon n.d.), focusing on women's reproductive role in relation to their children or fetus might lead to their disempowerment and justify a "growing surveillance on maternal conduct and intrusion into women's bodies" (Kimura 2013, 32).

Rediscovery is thus framed as an ongoing process to be completed. This is where promises come into play and offer new discursive resources to complete the expansion of amaranth cultivation and consumption.

Promissory Narratives

Many of our sources mention at least one promise that the rediscovery of amaranth could help fulfill. The most common is that of "alleviating/fighting/ tackling/combating" hunger, malnutrition, and obesity. Many of these promises build on war metaphors to frame the resurgence of amaranth as a strategy against hunger and malnutrition: "this plant is uniquely positioned in the fight against malnutrition" (López-Garcia 2008). Citing NGO staff members, a National Geographic article asserts that "bringing amaranth back into cultivation and consumption [will] help combat malnutrition" (Howard 2013). Following the classic structure of narratives (Adam 2005), amaranth promises have five components: initial situation, complication, reaction, resolution, and final solution. The path to solving the problem is dictated by the way the problem is framed. Since hidden hunger resulting from unbalanced diet has been framed as the main issue, and amaranth as a perfect combination of these valuable nutrients, how the resolution will take shape is self-evident. An author for *The Ecologist* asserts that "Oaxaca's rural communities survive on a very limited diet. This lack of diversity leads to deficiencies of amino acids and nutrients needed for growth, and can cause serious health problems" (Bruce 2014), while NGO Lexicon affirms that micronutrients present in amaranth[4] "are an incredibly important asset to strengthen diets, and particularly to prevent and treat malnourishment" (The Lexicon n.d.), this time using medical language. Citing NGO Puente's executive director, Al Jazeera journalist Kate Kilpatrick states that amaranth "has a unique fit into this enormous food crisis and health care crisis in Mexico" (Kilpatrick 2015). The revival of amaranth is therefore put forward as the one and only way to ensure a future where hunger and obesity will be defeated.

Promises are developed in connection with all the exceptional powers recognized for amaranth that we have already identified. Growing amaranth is presented as a path toward "adapting to" or "resisting" climate change, while as food it is deemed to have the power to "prevent" diseases (like cardiovascular diseases, birth defects, depression, or cancer). It could be used as well as an economic panacea to "reduce" or "address" poverty, "strengthen" regional economies, "improve" household food security and income, and "reduce" emigration. At last, as a relic of ancient civilizations, it would make it possible to "safeguard" traditions (Kilpatrick 2015), reactivate or reinvent cultural identities and social practices falling in disuse, revive biocultural heritage, including "native crops and cuisines" (Bruce 2014; Matsumoto 2017), and "promote" (agro)biodiversity. In this respect, amaranth is also recognized as conveying emancipatory power: "through reclaiming amaranth and traditional forms of cultivation and community organizing, rural communities are reclaiming their identity and sovereignty" (The Lexicon n.d.). Cultivating amaranth is expected to help farmers to "better connect to their roots" (Howard 2013) and to foster a "recovery of the traditional knowledge" (Slow Food 2007).

Most narratives of amaranth's deployment are not structured around a single promise but around bundles of promises, articulated by broad coalitions including food scientists (Venskutonis and Kraujalis 2013), NGOs (The Lexicon n.d.), and the media (Kilpatrick 2015). Various promises are piling up, thereby contributing to make the revival of amaranth cultivation and consumption an "obligatory passage point" (Akrich et al. 2006) to achieving desirable futures, just, prosperous, and climate resilient, free from hunger, obesity, disease, poverty, and deprivation. This echoes the findings of Rao and Huggins (2017) on biofortified sweet potato in Tanzania that promises of multiple "wins" as they call them go mainstream in the humanitarian and international development fields in response to donor expectations.

By definition, promissory narratives rely on idealized futures and on expectations that may fail to materialize. All the promises associated with the rediscovery of amaranth are based on vague allegations. They seldom refer to strong science-based evidence or verifiable sources beyond their endorsement by high-profile institutions like NASA or the World Health Organization that are reported to describe amaranth as a "well-balanced food" (Howard 2013). Yet these references can hardly be considered a scientific backing. They rather pertain to a type of "celebrity branding," that is, a marketing technique that uses the image and fame of the endorsers in hopes they will be passed on to the products, in this case the promise. The references to "studies" or "modern research" remain somewhat allusive: "studies have shown it to have cancer-preventing, anti-inflammatory and cholesterol-lowering properties"

(Kilpatrick 2015), or "modern research has discovered amaranth to have significant advantages over modern grains: it's easy to grow, easy to digest, and possesses superior nutrition" (Milner 2015). Whereas the virtues and powers of amaranth are forcefully asserted, these claims are neither based on numbers nor on measurements. For instance, amaranth is often claimed to have a high nutrient content, but no numbers are given. The voices of local experts (doctors, agronomists, nutritional experts) are called in as a pledge of integrity instead. They bring situated knowledge and field experience. This is part of a process of building the credibility and legitimacy of the promise. Finally, promises also make use of metaphors and other rhetoric devices that empower them.

Communication Style and Rhetoric Devices

The promises made around amaranth reflect the trend toward positive communication and the injunction associated with producing inspiring stories that drive hope instead of fear and focusing on "solutions" instead of problems (Nelder 2013). This trend is also present in the development aid sector where communication is moving away from despair and destitution to convey the struggles and hopes of local populations (Saillant et al. 2012), in order to arouse more positive emotions among donors. Communication scientists have indeed shown how the rhetoric of fear and catastrophe might end up being paralyzing and preventing action, whereas positive communication based on lexical fields of hope and love might conversely stimulate action (Nelder 2013). This is particularly visible in the documentation of the NGO Lexicon which aims at telling "inspiring" or "illuminating stories," "creating impact pathways," and "transforming lives" through "the contagiousness of hope" (The Lexicon n.d.). Likewise, journalists assert that "amaranth could be life changing" (Milner 2015), "creates the possibility of change" (Howard 2013), and "becomes a world of possibilities" (Del Moral 2017).

Along with its labeling as a "superfood," rediscovered amaranth is also depicted as a "powerful" crop or food by the media and (N)GOs. According to IFAD blog, amaranth has "super power" (Zins 2016) in that it "reduces cholesterol and can protect cells from cancer" while NGO Lexicon claims that amaranth and other "undervalued crops have the power to combat hunger" (The Lexicon n.d.). Amaranth is also compared by journalists to a nutritional "powerhouse" that can "boost" protein or folic acid intake. Others refer to the *poderes sobrenaturales* (El Correo del Sol n.d.) or assert that "Aztec believed that amaranth gave them physical and spiritual strength" (Milner 2015). But, as we have shown, the metaphors that fall within the lexical field of "fight" are the most frequent, mostly within claims to "fight" obesity and malnutrition or diseases. This is consistent with the findings of Breeze (2017) regarding medical and health claims related to superfoods.

A Not So New Framing

Based on this analysis, we could trace influences of the rediscovery discourse that merges various narratives and promises, namely the *Miracle Food* narrative (McDonell 2015), the *Slow Food* narrative (Petrini 2007), and especially the *Neglected and Under-utilized Species* (NUS) narrative (Rudebjer et al. 2014), recently rebranded as *Future Smart Food* narrative (Li and Siddique 2018). The NUS narrative emerged in the early 2000s under the impetus of the International Plant Genetic Resources Institute (IPGRI), now called Bioversity International, with the launch of a global initiative called "Neglected No More" in 2002 (see McDonell, this volume). The latter aimed at "contribut[ing] to raising the incomes and strengthening the food security of small farmers and rural communities around the world through securing and exploiting the full potential of the genetic diversity contained in neglected and underutilized species" (IPGRI 2002). Bioversity International thus appears as the main actor producing and diffusing the NUS narrative together with IFAD and the Food and Agriculture Organization (FAO). NUS, also referred to as "abandoned, lost, underused, local, minor, traditional, alternative, niche, or underdeveloped crops" (Padulosi 2017, 21), are first defined as plant species "to which little attention is paid or which are entirely ignored by agricultural researchers, plant breeders and policy makers"(Padulosi et al. 2013, 1) and that are "non-commodity crops" (Padulosi et al. 2013, 9). Their neglect and under-utilization are framed as both a cause and a consequence of an accelerated "loss" of diversity in food systems.

The NUS narrative sees the main cause of the abandonment of landraces in their exclusion from formal breeding programs that "has deprived underutilized crops of improved varieties" (Padulosi et al. 2013, 34) and has led to high production costs (Padulosi et al. 2014), which have resulted in the "underutilization" of those landraces. Therefore, solutions mainly focus on making the NUS "commercially attractive" (Clancy et al. n.d., 3) and breeding new varieties. This echoes the framing of the measures recommended to complete the rediscovery of amaranth.

The Untold Story

Following Hajer (2006), what the story tells might be as important as what it leaves out. A series of elements and protagonists of the rediscovery of amaranth is ignored in the proposed narrative, which results in significantly downplaying the complexity of the web of interests. For instance, the three NGO projects mentioned as success stories rely on multiple collaborations with international organizations like FAO, Slow Food, IFAD, research institutions both in Mexico and abroad, and national or international businesses like Kellogg's. These arrangements include direct funding and CSR, as well as commercial relationships (purchase of amaranth, distribution of cereal bars through NGO networks), and flows of knowledge and information.

Coloniality and modernization certainly played a critical role in the discarding of amaranth. Indeed, scholars have shown how the joint effects of the green revolution and the industrialization of food and food aid programs have helped impose the cultivation of improved Western varieties of cereals, the consumption of Western food, and even a neocolonial ontology of food as a fixed stock of nutrients (Peña et al. 2017) and crops as homogenous varieties (Demeulenaere 2014). Nevertheless, the latter are totally absent from the rediscovery narrative's apolitical framing of amaranth as a "forgotten" crop, rather than as a marginalized and subaltern crop. The rediscovery narrative even disseminates a neocolonial ontological representation of amaranth as a stock of (desirable) nutrients or (useful) genetic resources, whereas in a decolonial perspective it should be understood as having nurtured and been nurtured by communities (Peña et al. 2017) and as conveying affects as well as embodied cultural history (Aistara 2014). This highlights the persistence of neocolonial power structures (Pilcher 2012) and the colonization of mind (Mignolo 2009). According to Peña et al. (2017), a decolonization of food and diet should imply both a radical shift in the food system, breaking with what is termed the "imperialism" of the "neocolonial" agrochemical industry (Beilin and Suryanarayanan 2017, 206), and a decolonization of the representation of food. This would allow an increase in both social and epistemic justice, and to recognize both equality in diversity and diversity in equality (Santos 2011), but it does not seem to be the path taken by the rediscovery narrative.

As shown by McDonell (2015) in the case of quinoa, the "oblivion" might be exaggerated, as amaranth has never stopped being produced and consumed, but for self-consumption and in connection with particular social events that might have fallen under the radar of formal markets and official statistics (Katz and Lazos 2017). Anthropologists even claim there is a form of continuity in the cultivation, cultural uses, and knowledge of amaranth from precolonial times to the present in certain regions of Mexico (Velasco Lozano 2017; Villela Flores 2016). In such regions, scholars affirm that amaranth-related cultural practices "have resisted the assaults of evangelization and modernity and have supported ethnic identities" (Villela Flores 2016, 52, pers. trans.). Claiming amaranth was lost is a way to blur the active part played by farmers who have domesticated the plant and accompanied its evolution and adaptation over centuries through their breeding practices. This suggests that amaranth is a resource resulting from natural processes, discovered and valued by scientists, and denies its status as a product of patient breeding efforts over generations with obvious implications for the legitimacy granted to actors. The rediscovery narrative is centered on the plant and its powers, while the work and knowledge of farmers are made invisible. Farmers are considered in a paternalistic way as mere passive recipients of tools and expertise developed by external experts (scientists as well as NGOs) pushing further a process of de-skilling (Fitzgerald 1993), ultimately risking their alienation from seed and land.

Finally, the proposed framing of malnutrition, obesity, poverty, and the "loss" of agro-biodiversity is totally apolitical. This paves the way for the resolution of these problems through technical fixes. Accordingly, "natural" super-ancient food/crop and *ex situ* conservation are considered as such regardless of the broader political and institutional context of their deployment. For instance, the origin, legal, and genetic status of the seeds distributed by local NGOs as well as the intellectual property status envisaged for the future varieties are never mentioned. Nor is the fact that the three main collections of amaranth genetic resources to be used for breeding new varieties are found in gene banks outside Mexico, namely in the United States, India, and Peru (Joshi et al. 2018), and were established prior to the Convention on Biological Diversity and the Nagoya Protocol, and are therefore not subject to the access rules laid down in these texts.

Conclusion

The narrative of amaranth's rediscovery values it for its agronomic and nutritional qualities. It urges us to include amaranth into formal markets, research, and conservation systems to achieve the promised better futures. The rediscovery of amaranth and its recent consecration as a superfood seem to recycle and update preexisting discourses rather than being a real novelty.

As we have pointed out, the dominant narrative of this rediscovery gives some credit to indigenous communities of the past. It acknowledges and even exaggerates the historical injustice behind colonization by drawing upon unsubstantiated accounts of ban and punishment. By contrast, this narrative ignores the daily practices of production and consumption of amaranth among present-day indigenous communities and obscures the fact that they have never ceased to highlight the novelty of modern amaranth and its many promises. It also masks the neocolonial power relationship that has contributed to the marginalization of amaranth and its producers and disseminates a neocolonial ontological representation of amaranth as a stock of (desirable) nutrients or a set of (useful) genetic traits. Therefore, it pertains to the "fetishization of the (food) culture of ancient indigenous people" (Loyer and Knight 2018, 456) and to a form of "salvage capitalism" as defined by Anna Tsing (2015, 62) rather than to a decolonization process (Beilin and Suryanarayanan 2017).

Regardless of the power of this narrative, it does not follow that the revival of amaranth cultivation and consumption will uniformly follow the futures idealized for them. It cannot be inferred that Mexican peasants are irreparably reduced to the role of passive instruments in the expected amaranth boom. Research on techno-scientific promises and associated story lines has highlighted how unpredictable their effects can be (Joly 2013). As aptly expressed by Brown and Michael (2003, 7), "the past is littered with failed futures." Numerous examples also testify to the ability of farmers to divert, circumvent, and transform mainstream initiatives to their advantage (Van der Ploeg 2012). The micropolitics of amaranth rediscovery on the ground should therefore be thoroughly analyzed, which will be the next step in our research.

Notes

1   Nevertheless, "species number of amaranths is not certain because of gradual broadening of the gene pool due to frequent out crossing which has resulted in the emergence of a large number of varieties, morphotypes or cultivars with wide range of diversity, even species" (Das 2012, 273).

2   In a report titled "Underexploited Tropical Plants with Promising Economic Value," published in 1975.

3   *Puente a la Salud Communitaria* (Oaxaca) cited in nine publications, *Mexico Tierra de Amaranto* (Querretaro) cited in two publications, *Alternativas y Processos Sociales* (Puebla) cited in two publications.

4   Namely protein, lysine, fiber, calcium, iron, potassium, phosphorous, zinc, and vitamins A and C.

References

"Accelerated Food from the Sea Development Program" (1967), Box 12 folder 1, RG 22
　　Records concerning the Fish Protein Concentrate Program, 1959–68, US National
　　Archives and Records Administration.

Adam, J. M. (2005), *Les textes types et prototypes. Récit, description, argumentation,
　　explication et dialogue*, 2nd ed., Paris: Armand Colin.

Adhikari, M. (2005), *Not White Enough, Not Black Enough: Racial Identity in the South
　　African Coloured Community*, Africa Series, 83, Athens, OH: Ohio University Press.

Adhikari, M. (2010), "A Total Extinction Confidently Hoped For: The Destruction
　　of Cape San Society under Dutch Colonial Rule, 1700–1795," *Journal of Genocide
　　Research*, 12 (1–2): 19–44.

Aistara, G. (2014), "Actually Existing Tomatoes: Politics of Memory, Variety, and
　　Empire in Latvian Struggles over Seeds," *Focaal*, 69: 12–27. https://doi.org/10.3167/
　　fcl.2014.690102.

Akrich, M., M. Callon, and B. Latour (eds) (2006), *Sociologie de la traduction: Textes
　　fondateurs*, Paris: Presses de l'Ecole des Mines.

Albala, K. (2002), *Eating Right in the Renaissance*, Berkeley, CA: University of California
　　Press.

Alcázar, J. (1948), "Monografía de la quinua," *Boletin del Instituto Internacional
　　Americano de Protección a la Infancia*, 22: 357–69.

Allen, G. (2000), *The Almond People*. Sacramento, CA: Blue Diamond Growers.

Allen, G. (2018), "Employee Q&A: Dr. Karen Lapsley, Chief Scientific Officer," May
　　29, 2018. Available online: http://www.almonds.com/blog/employee-q-a-dr-karen-
　　lapsley-chief-scientific-officer.

Almond Board of California. (2018), "Snacking Tips," 2018. Available online: http://
　　www.almonds.com/consumers/snacking/snacking-tips.

Alvistur, E., P. White, and C. C. Chiriboga. (1953), "Biological Value of Quinoa," *Boletin
　　de la Sociedad Quimica del Peru*, 19: 197.

Alvord, S. H., L. D. Brown, and C. W. Letts. (2004), "Social Entrepreneurship and
　　Societal Transformation an Exploratory Study," *The Journal of Applied Behavioral
　　Science*, 40 (3): 260–82.

American Dietetic Association. (2009), "Position Statement on Functional Foods,"
　　2009. Available online: http://www.webdietitians.org/cps/rde/xchg/ada/hs.xsl/
　　advocacy_934_ENU_HTML.htm.

American Heart Association. (2018), "What's So Super about Superfoods?" Available
　　online: http://www.heart.org/HEARTORG/HealthyLiving/HealthyEating/Nutrition/
　　Whats-so-super-about-superfoods_UCM_457937_Article.jsp#.W1jSSNJKhPY
　　(accessed December 11, 2018).

Anderson, A. B., A. Gely, J. Strudwick, G. L. Sobel, and M. G. C. Pinto. (1985), "Um Sistema Agroforestal na Várzea do Estuário Amazônico (Ilha das Onças, Município de Barcarena, Estado do Pará)," *Acta Amazônica*, 15: 195–224.

Andina (2019), "Puno apuesta por la quinua orgánica para combatir anemia y desnutrición," *Empresa Peruana de Servicios Editoriales S. A. EDITORA*, May 21, 2019. Available online: https://andina.pe/agencia/noticia-puno-apuesta-por-quinua-organica-para-combatir-anemia-y-desnutricion-753002.aspx.

Andrews, L. B. (1996), "The Shadow Health Care System: Regulation of Alternative Health Care Providers," *Houston Law Review*, 32: 1273–317.

Appadurai, A. (1986), "Introduction: Commodities and the Politics of Value," in A. Appadurai (ed.), *The Social Life of Things: Commodities in Cultural Perspective*, 3–63, Cambridge, UK: Cambridge University Press.

Apple, R. (1996), *Vitamania: Vitamins in American Culture*, New Brunswick, NJ: Rutgers University Press.

Arai, S. (2002), "Global View on Functional Foods: Asian Perspectives," *British Journal of Nutrition*, 88 (Suppl. 2): S139–43.

Arévalo, A. F. and J. P. Maisch (eds) (1986), *Priorización y desarollo del sector agrario en el Perú*, Lima: Fundación Friedrich Ebert.

Ariel, A. (2012), "The Hummus Wars," *Gastronomica: The Journal of Critical Food Studies*, 12 (1): 34–42.

Atkins, P. (2010), *Liquid Materialities: A History of Milk, Science and the Law*, Surrey: Ashgate Press.

Atwater, W. O. (1895), "Food and Diet," US Department of Agriculture.

Balderas, O. (2018), "La revolución del amaranto," *Revista Cambio*, June 2018.

Barad, K. M. (2007), *Meeting the Universe Halfway: Quantum Physics and the Entanglement of Matter and Meaning*, Durham, NC: Duke University Press.

Basso, K. H. (1996), *Wisdom Sits in Places: Landscape and Language among the Western Apache*, Albuquerque, NM: University of New Mexico Press.

Bates, C. and C. Yerba. (1910), "They Came Three Thousand Miles to be with You at Christmas: California Soft-Shelled Almonds," UC Davis Special Collections.

Baudrillard, J. (1994), *Simulacra and Simulation*, Ann Arbor, MI: University of Michigan Press.

Bazile, D. (2014), "Estado del arte de la quinua en el mundo en 2013," FAO (Santiago de Chile) y CIRAD (Montpellier, Francia).

Bazile, D., S. E. Jacobsen, and A. Verniau. (2016), "The Global Expansion of Quinoa: Trends and Limits," *Frontiers in Plant Science*, 7: 622. https://doi.org/10.3389/fpls.2016.00622.

Beilin, K. and S. Suryanarayanan. (2017), "The War between Amaranth and Soy: Interspecies Resistance to Transgenic Soy Agriculture in Argentina," *Environmental Humanities*, 9 (2): 204–29. https://doi.org/10.1215/22011919-4215211.

Belasco, W. J. (2006), *Meals to Come: A History of the Future of Food*, Berkeley, CA: University of California Press.

Belasco, W. J. (2007), *Appetite for Change: How the Counterculture Took on the Food Industry*, 2nd updated ed., Ithaca, NY: Cornell University Press.

Benedictus, L. (2016), "The Truth about Superfoods," *The Guardian*, August 29, 2016. Available online: https://www.theguardian.com/lifeandstyle/2016/aug/29/truth-about-superfoods-seaweed-avocado-goji-berries-the-evidence.

Berkes, F. (1993), "Traditional Ecological Knowledge in Perspective," in J. T. Inglis (ed.), *Traditional Ecological Knowledge: Concepts and Cases*, 1–9, Ottawa: International Program on Traditional Ecological Knowledge and International Development Research Centre.

Berson, J. (2014), "The Quinoa Hack," *New Left Review*, 85: 117–32.

Besky, S. (2014), *The Darjeeling Distinction: Labor and Justice on Fair-Trade Tea Plantations in India*, Berkeley, CA: University of California Press.

Bezerra, V. S., O. Freitas-Silva, and L. F. Damasceno. (2016), "Açaí: producao de frutos, mercado e consume," *II Jornada Cientifica*. EMBRAPA.

Biltekoff, C. (2013), *Eating Right in America: The Cultural Politics of Food and Health/ Charlotte Biltekoff*, Durham, NC: Duke University Press.

Bitar, A. R. (2017), *Diet and the Disease of Civilization*. New Brunswick, NJ: Rutgers University Press.

Bittman, M. (2012), "The Right to Sell Kids Junk," *The New York Times: Opinion*, March 27, 2012. Available online: https://opinionator.blogs.nytimes.com/2012/03/27/the-right-to-sell-kids-junk/?_r=0.

Bobrow-Strain, A. (2011), "Making White Bread by the Bomb's Early Light: Anxiety, Abundance, and Industrial Food Power in the Early Cold War," *Food and Foodways*, 19 (1–2): 74–97.

Borup, M., N. Brown, K. Konrad, and V. L. Harro. (2006), "The Sociology of Expectations in Science and Technology," *Technology Analysis & Strategic Management*, 18 (3/4): 285–98. https://doi.org/10.1080/09537320600777002.

Boserup, E. (1965), *The Conditions of Agricultural Growth: The Economics of Agrarian Change under Population Pressure*, Chicago, IL: Aldine.

Bourdieu, P. (1971), "Le marche des biens symboliques," *L'Année sociologique*, 22 (49–126): 1971.

Boyd, S. (2018), "How This Couple Launched Their Health-Focused Business," *Forbes*, May 31. Available online: https://www.forbes.com/sites/sboyd/2018/05/31/your-super/#569946f46c26.

Boyland, E. J., S. Nolan, B. Kelly, C. Tudur-Smith, A. Jones, J. C. Halford, and E. Robinson. (2016), "Advertising as a Cue to Consume: A Systematic Review and Meta-Analysis of the Effects of Acute Exposure to Unhealthy Food and Nonalcoholic Beverage Advertising on Intake in Children and Adults," *American Journal of Clinical Nutrition*, 103 (2): 519–33. https://doi.org/10.3945/ajcn.115.120022.

Bracker, M. (1948), Latin Nations See New Food in Quinoa, U.N. Group to Study Nutritive Value of Ancient Inca Plant for Upland Indigenes 10.

Breeze, R. (2017), "Explaining Superfoods: Exploring Metaphor Scenarios in Media Science Reports," *Ibérica: Revista de la Asociación Europea de Lenguas para Fines Específicos (AELFE)*, 67–88.

British Nutrition Foundation. (2017), "Tomatoes Grow Underground and Pasta Comes from Animals, According to UK School Children and Teens." Available online: https://www.nutrition.org.uk/press-office/pressreleases/1059-bnfhew2017.html.

Brondizio, E. S. (2004), "From Staple to Fashion Food: Shifting Cycles, Shifting Opportunities in the Development of the Açaí Fruit (Euterpe oleracea Mart.) Economy in the Amazon Estuary," in D. Zarin (ed.), *Working Forests in the American Tropics: Conservation through Sustainable Management?* 348–61, New York: Columbia University Press.

Brondizio, E. S. (2008), *Amazonian Caboclo and the Acai Palm: Forest Farmers in the Global Market*, New York: New York Botanical Garden Press.

Brondizio, E. S. (2011), "Forest Resources, Family Networks and the Municipal Disconnect: Examining Recurrent Underdevelopment in the Amazon Estuary," in M. Pinedo-Vasquez, M. M. Ruffino, C. Padoch, and E. S. Brondizio (eds), *The Amazonian Várzea: The Decade Past and the Decade Ahead*, 207–32, Dordrecht, The Netherlands: Springer Publishers Co-publication with The New York Botanical Garden Press.

Brondizio, E. S. and A. D. Siqueira. (1997), "From Extractivists to Forest Farmers: Changing Concepts of Caboclo Agroforestry in the Amazon Estuary," *Research in Economic Anthropology*, 18: 234–79.

Brondizio, E. S., N. Vogt, and A. Siqueira. (2013), "Forest Resources, City Services: Globalization, Household Networks, and Urbanization in the Amazon Estuary," in K. Morrison, S. Hetch and C. Padoch (eds), *The Social Life of Forests*, 348–61, Chicago, IL: The University of Chicago Press.

Brown, W. (2003), "Neo-Liberalism and the End of Liberal Democracy," *Theory & Event*, 7 (1): 3–18.

Brown, N. and M. Michael. (2003), "A Sociology of Expectations: Retrospecting Prospects and Prospecting Retrospects," *Technology Analysis & Strategic Management*, 15 (1): 3–18. https://doi.org/10.1080/0953732032000046024.

Bruce, A. (2014), "Amaranth Revival—Mexican Farmers Rediscover an Ancient Superfood," *The Ecologist*, October 25, 2014.

Burwood-Taylor, L. (2017), *Eighteen94 Capital Leads Funding in Kuli Kuli*. Available online: https://agfundernews.com/breaking-kelloggs-vc-1894-capital-makes-first-investment-agfunder-alum-kuli-kuli.html.

Butler, C. and J. Holston ([1966]), "Man's Key Protein Awaits Harvest from the Sea," Box 1 FPC Correspondence file 6 March–August 66, RG 22 Records concerning the Fish Protein Concentrate Program, 1959–1968, US National Archives and Records Administration.

CABI. (2019), *Moringa oleifera (Horse Radish Tree)*. CABI Invasive Species Compendium. Available online: https://www.cabi.org/isc/datasheet/34868.

Calderon, C. (2017), "Six Latino 'Superfoods' You Should Add to Your Diet," *NBC News*.

Campbell, A. J., L. G. Carvalheiro, M. M. Maués et al. (2018), "Anthropogenic Disturbance of Tropical Forests Threatens Pollination Services to Açaí Palm in the Amazon River Delta," *Journal of Applied Ecology*, 2018 (55): 1725–36. https://doi.org/10.1111/1365-2664.13086.

Cao, G. (1997), "Antioxidant and Prooxidant Behavior of Flavonoids: Structure-Activity Relationships," *Free Radical Biology and Medicine*, 22 (5): 749–60.

Cao, G., H. M. Alessio, and R. G. Cutler. (1993), "Oxygen-Radical Absorbance Capacity Assay for Antioxidants," *Free Radical Biology and Medicine*, 14: 303–11.

Cao, G., E. Sofic, and R. L. Prior. (1996), "Antioxidant Capacity of Tea and Common Vegetables," *Journal of Agricultural and Food Chemistry*, 44: 3426–31.

Cao, G., C. P. Verdon, A. H. Wu, H. Wang, and R. L. Prior. (1995), "Automated Assay of Oxygen Radical Absorbance Capacity with the COBAS FARA II," *Clinical Chemistry*, 41 (12): 1738–44.

Carolan, M. S. (2011), *Embodied Food Politics*, New York: Ashgate.

Carpenter, K. J. (1994), *Protein and Energy: A Study of Changing Ideas in Nutrition*, Cambridge: Cambridge University Press.

Castree, N. and B. Braun (1998), "The Construction of Nature and the Nature of Construction," in N. Castree and B. Braun (eds), *Remaking Nature: Nature and the Millennium*, 3–32, London: Routledge.

Center for Food Safety and Applied Nutrition, Office of Nutritional Products, Labeling, and Dietary Supplements. (2013), "A Food Labeling Guide: Guidance for Industry," *U.S. Department of Health and Human Services*. Available online: www.fda.gov/foodlabelingguide.

Cernansky, R. (2015), "The Rise of Africa's Super Vegetables," *Nature News*, 522: 146–8. https://doi.org/10.1038/522146a.

Chatterjee, P. (2001), *A Time for Tea: Women, Labor, and Post/colonial Politics on an Indian Plantation*. Durham, NC: Duke University Press.

Chennells A. (2010), Letter to the Director General, Department Water and Environmental Affairs.

Chera, M. (2020), Tamil Traditions: Women Cooking and Eating for Heritage and Health in South India, Ph.D. Dissertation, Indiana University Bloomington.

Chernev, A. (2011), "The Dieter's Paradox," *Journal of Consumer Psychology*, 21 (2): 178–83. https://doi.org/10.1016/j.jcps.2010.08.002.

Cho, A. H. (2006), "Politics, Values and Social Entrepreneurship: A Critical Appraisal," in J. Mair, J. Robinson and K. Hockerts (eds), *Social Entrepreneurship*, 34–56, London: Palgrave Macmillan UK.

Clancy, E., R. Vernooy, A. Drucker, J. van Etten, A. Gupta, M. Halewood, D. Jarvis, R. Nankya, I. L. Noriega, S. Padulosi, M. Ramírez, N. Sharma, and B. Sthapit. (n.d.), *Realizing Farmers' Rights through Community-Based Agricultural Biodiversity Management*. Rome: Bioversity International.

Clark, A. E., L. Mamo, J. R. Fosket, J. R. Fishman, and J. K. Shim (eds) (2010), *Biomedicalization: Technoscience, Health, and Illness in the U.S.*, Durham, NC: Duke University Press.

Cobb Bates & Yerba Co. (1910), "They Came Three Thousand Miles to be with You at Christmas: California Soft-Shelled Almonds," UC Davis Special Collections.

Cochrane, W. W. (1993), *The Development of American Agriculture: A Historical Analysis*, 2nd ed., Minneapolis, MN: University of Minnesota Press.

Coles, B. (2016), "The Shocking Materialities and Temporalities of Agri-Capitalism," *Gastronomica: The Journal of Critical Food Studies*, 16 (3): 5–12. https://doi.org/10.1525/gfc.2016.16.3.5.

Collins, J. (2014), "A Feminist Approach to Overcoming the Closed Boxes of the Commodity Chain," in W. Dunaway (ed.), *Gendered Commodity Chains*, 27–37, Stanford, CA: Stanford University Press.

"Colorful Foods: The Benefits of Eating the Rainbow" (2017), Swissôtel Hotels & Resorts. Available online: http://www.swissotel.com/infographics/eat-a-rainbow/.

Comptroller General of the United States. (1973), "Fish Protein Concentrate Program." Available online: www.gao.gov/assets/210/203766.pdf.

"Conversation with Dr. Weinberg of the Ministry of Industry, Canada on May 11, 1967" (1967), Box 2 folder 1, RG 22 Records concerning the Fish Protein Concentrate Program, 1959–1968, US National Archives and Records Administration.

Cook, I. and P. Crang. (1996), "The World on a Plate: Culinary Culture, Displacement and Geographical Knowledge," *Journal of Material Culture*, 1: 131–53.

Coombe, R. J., S. Ives, and D. Huizenga. (2015), "The Social Imaginary of Geographical Indicators in Contested Environments: The Politicized Heritage and the Racialized Landscapes of South African Rooibos Tea," in M. David and D. Halbert (eds), *The Sage Handbook of Intellectual Property*, 224–37, London: Sage.

Costa, F. A. (2016), *O Açaí do Grão-Pará: Arranjos Produtivos e Economia Local— Estruturação e Dinâmica (1995–2011), Tese de livre docencia*. Belem: Universidade Federal do Para (UFPA).

Cravioto, J., E. R. DeLicardie, and H. G. Birch. (1966), "Nutrition, Growth and Neurointegrative Development: An Experimental and Ecological Study," *Pediatrics*, 38 (2): 319–20.

Crawford, E. (2018), *Kuli Kuli Explains Why Its Growing Portfolio of Moringa Products is Worth More than the Competition*. Available online: https://www.foodnavigator-usa.com/Article/2018/07/12/Kuli-Kuli-explains-why-its-growing-portfolio-of-moringa-products-is-worth-more-than-the-competition?utm_source=copyright&utm_medium=OnSite&utm_campaign=copyright.

Crawford, E. (2019), "Your Super Raises $5M to Introduce the Power of Superfoods to More Americans," *Food Navigator USA*, January 31. Available online: https://www.foodnavigator-usa.com/Article/2019/01/31/Your-Super-raises-5M-to-introduce-the-power-of-superfoods-to-more-Americans.

Crawford, R. (2006), "Health as a Meaningful Social Practice," *Health*, 10 (4): 401–20.

Cullather, N. (2010), *The Hungry World: America's Cold War Battle against Poverty in Asia*, Cambridge: Harvard University Press.

Culley, W. J. (1975), "Nutrition and Mental Retardation," in C. H. Carter (ed.), *Medical Aspects of Mental Retardation*, 73–82, Springfield, IL: Charles C. Thomas Publisher.

Curll, J., C. Parker, C. MacGregor, and A. Peterson. (2016), "Unlocking the Energy of the Amazon? The Need for a Food Fraud Policy Approach to the Regulation of Anti-Aging Health Claims on Superfood Labelling," *Federal Law Review*, 44: 419–49.

Curtis, L. (2019), *Lisa Curtis*. LinkedIn. Available online: https://www.linkedin.com/in/lisamariecurtis.

Cusack, D. (1984), "Quinoa: Grain of the Incas," *The Ecologist*, 14: 21–3.

Cutler, H. C. (1954), "Food Sources in the New World," *Agricultural History*, 28: 43–9.

Darby, M. R. and E. Karni. (1973), "Free Competition and the Optimal Amount of Fraud," *The Journal of Law and Economics*, 16 (1): 67–88.

Das, S. (2012), "Domestication, Phylogeny and Taxonomic Delimitation in Underutilized Grain *Amaranthus* (Amaranthaceae)—A Status Review," *Feddes Repertorium*, 123: 273–82. https://doi.org/10.1002/fedr.201200017.

Davis, F. (1992), *Fashion, Culture, and Identity*. Chicago, IL: University of Chicago Press.

Day, P. and C. Steyeart. (2012), "Social Entrepreneurship: Critique and the Radical Enactment of the Social," *Social Enterprise Journal*, 9: 90–107.

De Shield, C. (2015), "The Cosmopolitan Amaranth: A Postcolonial Ecology," *Postcolonial Text*, 10 (1).

Deighton, N., R. Brennan, C. Finn, and H. Davies. (2000), "Antioxidant Properties of Domesticated and Wild Rubus Species," *Journal of the Science of Food and Agriculture*, 3, 80 (9): 1307–13.

Del Moral, S. (2017), "El amaranto, la alegría de la agricultura Mexicana," *Vice Mexico*, June 2017.

Demeulenaere, E. (2014), "A Political Ontology of Seeds. The Transformative Frictions of a Farmers' Movement in Europe," *Focaal*, 69: 45–61. https://doi.org/10.3167/fcl.2014.690104.

Department of Environmental Affairs. (2014), *Traditional Knowledge Associated with Rooibos and Honeybush Species in South Africa*. Available online: https://www.environment.gov.za/otherdocuments/reports.

Diener, P., K. Moore, and R. Mutaw. (1980), "Meats, Markets, and Mechanical Materialism: The Great Protein Fiasco in Anthropology," *Dialectical Anthropology*, 5 (3): 171–92.

Dietler, M. (2006), "Culinary Encounters: Food, Identity, and Colonialism," in K. C. Twiss (ed.), *The Archaeology of Food and Identity, Center for Archaeological Investigations*, 218–42, Carbondale: Southern Illinois University.

Dixon, J. (2009), "From the Imperial to the Empty Calorie: How Nutrition Relations Underpin Food Regime Transitions," *Agriculture and Human Values*, 26 (4): 321–33. https://doi.org/10.1007/s10460-009-9217-6.

Dixon, J. and C. Banwell. (2004), "Re-Embedding Trust: Unravelling the Construction of Modern Diets," *Critical Public Health*, 14 (2): 117–31. https://doi.org/10.1080/09581590410001725364.

Dixon, J., L. Hattersley, and B. Isaacs. (2014), "Transgressing Retail: Supermarkets, Liminoid Power and the Metabolic Rift," in M. K. Goodman and C. Sage (eds), *Food Transgressions: Making Sense of Contemporary Food Politics*, 131–54, London: Ashgate.

Doeppers, D. F. (2016), *Feeding Manila in Peace and War, 1850–1945*. Madison, WI: University of Wisconsin Press.

Dohrenwend, A. S. (2019), "Socio-Environmental Impacts of Argentine Yerba Mate Cultivation: 'El Problema es el Precio Bajo,'" Thesis, University of Kansas.

Dolan, C. (2012), "The New Face of Development: The 'Bottom of the Pyramid' Entrepreneurs," *Anthropology Today*, 28 (4): 3–7.

Dolan, C. S. (2010), "Virtual Moralities: The Mainstreaming of Fairtrade in Kenyan Tea Fields," *Geoforum*, 41 (1): 33–43.

Dolan, C. S. (2014), "Business as a Development Agent: Evidence of Possibility and Improbability," *Third World Quarterly*, 35 (1): 22–42. https://doi.org/10.1080/014365 97.2013.868982.

Dove, M. (2011), *The Banana Tree at the Gate: A History of Marginal Peoples and Global Markets in Borneo*, New Haven, CT: Yale University Press.

Dreher, M. (2017), "Almonds and Wellness," *California Almonds: Newsroom* (blog), 2017. Available online: http://newsroom.almonds.com/index.php/content/almonds-and-wellness-mark-dreher-chairman-nutrition-research-committee.

Dreher, N. (2018), "Food from Nowhere: Complicating Cultural Food Colonialism to Understand Matcha as Superfood," *Graduate Journal of Food Studies*, 5.

Drew, J., A. D. Sachs, C. Sueiro, and J. R. Stepp. (2017), "Ancient Grains and New Markets: The Selling of Quinoa as Story and Substance," in *Corporate Social Responsibility and Corporate Governance, Developments in Corporate Governance and Responsibility*, vol. 11, 251–74, Emerald Publishing Limited, https://doi.org/10.1108/S2043-052320170000011012.

Dumit, J. (2012), *Drugs for Life: How Pharmaceutical Companies Define Our Health*, Durham, NC: Duke University Press.

DuPuis, E. M. (2002), *Nature's Perfect Food: How Milk Became America's Drink*, New York: New York University Press.

DuPuis, E. M. (2015), *Dangerous Digestion: The Politics of American Dietary Advice*, Berkeley, CA: University of California Press.

Earle, R. (2014), *The Body of the Conquistador*, Cambridge: Cambridge University Press.

Early, D. (1992), "The Renaissance of Amaranth," in N. Foster and L. S. Cordell (eds), *Chilies to Chocolate: Food the Americas Gave the World*, 15–34, Tucson: The University of Arizona Press.

Eaton, S. (2013), "Alt Staple Lunch: Mexicans Push Return of an Ancient Grain," *The World*, July 2013.

Ebrahim, S. (2016), "Science Has Proven It—Rooibos Tea Is Magic," *The Daily Vox*. Available online: https://www.thedailyvox.co.za/science-proven-rooibos-tea-magic/.

Eglash, R. (2013), "Technology as Material Culture," in C. Y. Tilley (ed.), *Handbook of Material Culture*, 1. pbk. ed., 329–40, London: Sage.

Egoávil, M., J. Reinoso, and H. A. Torres. (1979), *Fomento de la producción agroindustrial de Quinua en el Departamento de Puno: Análisis de los costos y canales de comercialización de la quinua, Fondo Simon Bolivar*, Lima: Universidad Nacional Técnca del Altiplano.

Ehlenfeldt, M. K. and R. L. Prior. (2001), "Oxygen Radical Absorbance Capacity (ORAC) and Phenolic and Anthocyanin Concentrations in Fruit and Leaf Tissues of Highbush Blueberry," *Journal of Agricultural and Food Chemistry*, 49: 2222–7.

Eiselen, E. (1956), "Quinoa, a Potentially Important Food Crop of the Andes," *Journal of Geography*, 55: 330–3. https://doi.org/10.1080/00221345608983004.

El Correo del Sol. (n.d.), "Amaranto, el gran secreto de los Incas," *El Correo del Sol*.

Elbein, S. (2013), "The Seeds That Time Forgot," *The Texas Observer*, 105 (April): 26–9.

Elmer, L. A. (1942), "Quinoa (Chenopodium quinoa)," *East African Agricultural Journal*, 8: 21–3. https://doi.org/10.1080/03670074.1942.11664212.

Ensminger, A. H., M. E. Ensminger, J. E. Konlande, and J. R. K. Robson. (1994), "Eggs, Dehydrated," in *Foods & Nutrition Encyclopedia*, vol. 1, 2nd ed., 645–6, New York: Chemical Rubber Company Press.

Espitia Rangel, E. (2016), "Etnología del amaranto," *Arqueología Mexicana*, 138: 64–70.

"Everything Changed after My Cancer Diagnosis at Age 24" (n.d.), *Your Super Email Newsletter* (received March 28, 2019).

Falk, P. (1994), *The Consuming Body*, London: Sage Publications.

FAO (2013), "Launch of the International Year of Quinoa." February 20, 2013. http://www.fao.org/quinoa-2013/press-room/news/detail/en/.

FAO (2018), "Once Neglected, These Traditional Crops Are Our New Rising Stars." Food and Agriculture Organization of the United Nations. February 10, 2018. http://www.fao.org/fao-stories/article/en/c/1154584/.

Farquhar, J. (2002), *Appetites: Food and Sex in Post-Socialist China*, Durham, NC: Duke University Press.

Feldman, A. (2017), *A Startup Backed by Kellogg's VC Arm, Kuli Kuli, Introduces Americans to a New Superfood, Moringa*. Available online: https://www.forbes.com/sites/forbestreptalks/2017/10/05/a-startup-backed-by-kelloggs-vc-arm-kuli-kuli-introduces-americans-to-a-new-superfood-moringa/#3cb366b64e06.

Ferguson, J. (1990), *The Anti-Politics Machine*, New York: Cambridge University Press.

Fernandez, D. G. (1994), *Tikim: Essays on Philippine Food and Culture*. Pasig City, Philippines: Anvil Publishing.

Fernandez, D. G. and E. N. Alegre. (1988), *Sarap: Essays on Philippine Food*. Manila, Philippines: Mr. and Ms Publishing Company.

Ferroni, M. A. (1982), "Food Habits and the Apparent Nature and Extent of Dietary Nutritional Deficiencies in the Peruvian Andes," *Archives Latino-americanos de Nutrición*, 32: 850–66.

Field, R. C. (2000), "Cruciferous and Green Leafy Vegetables," in K. F. Kiple (ed.), *The Cambridge World History of Food*, 288–98, Cambridge, UK: Cambridge University Press.

Filley, H. C. (1929), *Cooperation in Agriculture*, New York: John Wiley & Sons, Inc.

Finnis, E. (ed.) (2012), *Reimagining Marginalized Foods: Global Processes, Local Places*, Tucson, AZ: University of Arizona Press.

Fischer, E. F. and P. Benson. (2006), *Broccoli and Desire: Global Connections and Maya Struggles in Postwar Guatemala*, Stanford, CA: Stanford University Press.

"Fish Protein Concentrate" (1966), Box 1 FPC Correspondence file August 5, 1965–February 1966, RG 22 Records concerning the Fish Protein Concentrate Program, 1959–1968, US National Archives and Records Administration.

Fitzgerald, D. (1993), "Farmers Deskilled: Hybrid Corn and Farmers' Work," *Technology and Culture*, 34: 324–43. https://doi.org/10.2307/3106539.

Fleischmann, E. and L. Muir. (2018), "Almonds in the Global Marketplace," Presentation presented at the Almond Conference, Sacramento, CA, USA, December 4. Available online: http://www.almonds.com/sites/default/files/content/attachments/Almonds%20in%20the%20Global%20Marketplace.pdf.

Food from the Sea Service, Office of the War on Hunger (1967), "Food from the Sea: A Demonstration Program for Latin America," Box 12 folder 2, RG 22 Records concerning the Fish Protein Concentrate Program, 1959–1968, US National Archives and Records Administration.

Foss, R. (2015), *Food in the Air and Space: The Surprising History of Food and Drink in the Skies*, New York: Rowman & Littlefield.

Foster, L. A. (2017), *Reinventing Hoodia: Peoples, Plants, and Patents in South Africa*, Seattle, WC: University of Washington Press.

Foucault, M. (1988), *Technologies of the Self: A Seminar with Michel Foucault*, edited by L. H. Martin, H. Gutman, and P. H. Hutton. Amherst, MA: University of Massachusetts Press.

Foucault, M. (1990 [1978]), *The History of Sexuality, Vol. 1: An Introduction*, New York: Vintage.

Foyer, Jean, Aurore Viard-Crétat et Valérie Boisvert. (2017), "Néolibéraliser sans marchandiser? La bioprospection et les mécanismes REDD dans l'économie de la promesse," in D. Compagnon and E. Rodary (eds), *Les politiques de biodiversité*, 225–49, Paris: Presses de Sciences Po.

Freidberg, S. (2004), *French Beans and Food Scares: Culture and Commerce in an Anxious Age*, New York: Oxford University Press.

Friedmann, H. (1993), "The Political Economy of Food," *New Left Review*, 197: 29–57.

GAO. (1985), "The Role of Marketing Orders in Establishing and Maintaining Orderly Marketing Conditions," GAO/RCED-85-57. United States General Accounting Office.

García, M. E. (2010), Super Guinea Pigs? *Anthropology Now*, 2: 22–32.

García, M. E. (2013), "The Taste of Conquest: Colonialism, Cosmopolitics, and the Dark Side of Peru's Gastronomic Boom," *The Journal of Latin American and Caribbean Anthropology*, 18 (3): 505–24. https://doi.org/10.1111/jlca.12044.

Gillon, S. (2016), "Flexible for Whom? Flex Crops, Crises, Fixes and the Politics of Exchanging Use Values in US Corn Production," *The Journal of Peasant Studies*, 43 (1): 117–39. https://doi.org/10.1080/03066150.2014.996555.

Gilman, N. (2003), *Mandarins of the Future: Modernization Theory in Cold War America*, Baltimore, MD: Johns Hopkins University Press.

"Giving Back" (n.d.), *Your Super*. Available online: https://yoursuper.com/pages/givingback.

Glover, D. and G. D. Stone. (2018), "Heirloom Rice in Ifugao: An 'Anti-commodity' in the Process of Commodification," *The Journal of Peasant Studies*, 45 (4): 776–804.

Goldstein, J. (2018), *Planetary Improvement: Cleantech Entrepreneurship and the Contradictions of Green Capitalism*. Cambridge, MA: MIT Press.

Gómez, F. (1961), "The Use of Fish Flour in Human Nutrition," *Boletín Médico del Hospital Infantil de México*, 1 (1), Box 7 "FDA Fish Flour Background Information," RG 22 Records concerning the Fish Protein Concentrate Program, 1959–1968, National Archives and Records Administration.

Goodman, M. K. (2004), "Reading Fair Trade: Political Ecological Imaginary and the Moral Economy of Fair Trade Foods," *Political Geography*, 23 (7): 891–915.

Gorelik, B. (2017), *Rooibos: An Ethnographic Perspective*, Rooibos Council. Available online: https://sarooibos.co.za/rooibos-an-ethnographic-perspective/ (accessed December 12, 2018).

Graddy-Lovelace, G. and A. Diamond. (2017), "From Supply Management to Agricultural Subsidies—And Back Again? The U.S. Farm Bill & Agrarian (in)Viability," *Journal of Rural Studies*, 50 (February): 70–83. https://doi.org/10.1016/j.jrurstud.2016.12.007.

Grand View Research. (2016), "Argan Oil Market Size, Share & Trends Analysis Report by Application (Cosmetics, Food, Medical), by Region (North America, Europe, Asia Pacific, Middle & East Africa, Central & South America), and Segment Forecasts, 2015–2022," Market Research Report. Available online: https://www.grandviewresearch.com/industry-analysis/argan-oil-market.

Grasseni, C., H. Paxson, A. J. Jim Bingen, S. F. Cohen, and H. G. West. (2014), "Introducing a Special Issue on the Reinvention of Food Connections and Mediations," *Gastronomica: The Journal of Critical Food Studies*, 14 (4): 1–6.

Greene, S. (2004), "Indigenous People Incorporated? Culture as Politics, Culture as Property in Pharmaceutical Bioprospecting," *Current Anthropology*, 45: 211–37. https://doi.org/10.1086/381047.

Groeniger, J. O., F. J. v. Lenthe, M. A. Beenackers, and B. M. K. Carlijn. (2017), "Does Social Distinction Contribute to Socioeconomic Inequalities in Diet?: The Case of 'Superfoods' Consumption," *International Journal of Behavioral Nutrition and Physical Activity*, 14 (40).

Grose, J. (2011), "Rooibos Tea: If You Haven't Heard of It, You Will Soon," *Slate*. Available online: http://www.slate.com/articles/life/drink/2011/06/rooibos_tea.html.

Guardino, M. and D. Snyder. (2017), "The Capitalist Advertising and Marketing Complex and the US Social Order: A Political-Materialist Analysis," *New Political Science*, 39 (4): 588–608. https://doi.org/10.1080/07393148.2017.1379736.

Guest. (2019), *Kuli Kuli on Diversifying Monocultures of People and Plants*. Available online: https://foodtechconnect.com/2019/01/10/kuli-kuli-on-diversifying-monocultures-of-people-and-plants/?mc_cid=bd9e6831ee&mc_eid=f9b8ec1b37.

Guthman, J. (2003), "Fast Food/Organic Food: Reflexive Tastes and the Making of 'Yuppie Chow,'" *Social & Cultural Geography*, 4: 45–58.

Guthman, J. (2004), "The 'Organic Commodity' and Other Anomalies in the Politics of Consumption," in A. Hughes and S. Reimer (eds), *Geographies of Commodity Chains*, 233–49, London: Routledge.

Guthman, J. (2008), "Neoliberalism and the Making of Food Politics in California," *Geoforum*, 39 (3): 1171–83. https://doi.org/10.1016/j.geoforum.2006.09.002.

Guthman, J. (2009), "Unveiling the Unveiling: Commodity Chains, Commodity Fetishism, and the 'Value' of Voluntary, Ethical Food Labels," in J. Bair (ed.), *Frontiers of Commodity Chain Research*, 190–206, Stanford, CA: Stanford University Press.

Guthman, J. (2011), *Weighing In: Obesity, Food Justice, and the Limits of Capitalism*, Berkeley, CA: University of California Press.

Guthman, J. (2015), "Binging and Purging: Agrofood Capitalism and the Body as Socioecological Fix," *Environment and Planning A*, 47 (12): 2522–36. https://doi.org/10.1068/a140005p.

Guthman, J. and M. DuPuis. (2006), "Embodying Neoliberalism: Economy, Culture, and the Politics of Fat," *Environment and Planning D: Society and Space*, 24 (3): 427–48. https://doi.org/10.1068/d3904.

Hajer, M. (2006), "Doing Discourse Analysis: Coalitions, Practices, Meaning," in M. van den Brink and T. Metze (eds), *Words Matter in Policy and Planning: Discourse Theory and Method in the Social Sciences*, 65–74, Utrecht: NGS/KNAG/Nethur Netherland Geographical Institute.

Hajer, M. and W. Versteeg. (2005), "A Decade of Discourse Analysis of Environmental Politics: Achievements, Challenges, Perspectives," *Journal of Environmental Policy and Planning*, 7 (3): 175–84.

Hall, K. Q. (2014), "Toward a Queer Crip Feminist Politics of Food," *philoSOPHIA*, 4 (2): 177–96.

Hamada, S. and R. Wilk. (2019), *Seafood: Ocean to the Plate*, New York: Routledge.

Hancock, R. D., G. J. McDougall, and D. Stewart. (2007), "Berry Fruit as 'Superfood': Hope or Hype?" *Biologist*, 54: 73–9.

Hanna, S. (2012), *The Book of Kale: The Easy to Grow Superfood*. Madeira Park, BC: Harbour Publishing.

"Happy Customers" (n.d.), *Your Super*. Available online: https://yoursuper.com/pages/happy-customers.

Haraway, D. (1997), *Modest Witness@Second Millennium*, New York: Routledge.

Haraway, D. J. (1991), *Simians, Cyborgs, and Women: The Reinvention of Nature*, New York: Routledge.

Harding, S. (1986), *The Science Question in Feminism*, Cornell, NY: Cornell University Press.

Harvey, D. (1981), "The Spatial Fix–Hegel, von Thunen, and Marx," *Antipode*, 13 (3): 1–12.

Harvey, D. (2001), "Globalization and the Spatial Fix," *Geographische Revue*, 2 (3): 23–31.

Harvey, D. (2006), *The Limits to Capital*. London; New York: Verso.

Hasler, C. M. (2002), "Functional Foods: Benefits, Concerns and Challenges—A Position Paper from the American Council on Science and Health," *The Journal of Nutrition*, 132 (12): 3772–81. https://doi.org/10.1093/jn/132.12.3772.

Hayden, C. (2003), *When Nature Goes Public: The Making and Unmaking of Bioprospecting in Mexico*, Princeton, NJ: Princeton University Press.

Hayes-Conroy, A. and J. Hayes-Conroy (eds) (2013), *Doing Nutrition Differently: Critical Approaches to Diet and Dietary Intervention*, New York: Routledge.

Haytowitz, D. B. and S. Bhagwat. (2010), "USDA Database for the Oxygen Radical Absorbance Capacity (ORAC) of Selected Foods, Release 2," U.S. Department of Agriculture, Agricultural Research Service. Available online: http://www.ars.usda.gov/nutrientdata/orac.

Heller, I. R. (2005), "Functional Foods: Regulatory and Marketing Developments in the United States," in C. M. Hasler (ed.), *Regulation of Functional Food and Nutraceuticals*, 169–99, Ames, IA: Blackwell Press.

Helms, M. W. (1988), *Ulysses' Sail: An Ethnographic Odyssey of Power, Knowledge, and Geographical Distance*, Princeton, NJ: Princeton University Press.

Henshall, S. (2012), "What Causes Boom and Bust?" *Socialist Review*. http://socialistreview.org.uk/368/what-causes-boom-and-bust.

Hiraoka, M. (1994), "Mudanças nos Padrões Econômicos de uma População Ribeirinha do Estuário do Amazonas," in L. Furtado, A. F. Mello and W. Leitão (eds), *Povos das Águas: Realidade e Perspectivas na Amazônia*, 133–57, Belém: MPEG/Universidade Federal do Pará.

Hobart, H. (2017), "A 'Queer-Looking Compound': Race, Abjection, and the Politics of Hawaiian Poi," *Global Food History*, 3 (2): 133–49. https://doi.org/10.1080/20549547.2017.1352441.

Hoffman, I. (2003), "Transcending Reductionism in Nutrition Research," *The American Journal of Clinical Nutrition*, 78 (3): 5145–65.

Howard, B. (2013), "Amaranth: Another Ancient Wonder Food, but Who Will Eat it?" *National Geographic* August 10, 12, 2013.

Huang, D., B. Ou, and R. L. Prior. (2005), "The Chemistry behind Antioxidant Capacity Assays," *Journal of Agricultural and Food Chemistry*, 53: 1841–56.

Huwyler, N. (2016), "Les superaliments: Une révolution ou un mythe?" *Tabula*, 1: 4–7.

IBGE. (2017), "Censo Agropecuario," Instituto Brasileira de Geografia e Estatistica 2017. Available online: https://sidra.ibge.gov.br/pesquisa/censo-agropecuario/censo-agropecuario-2017

IBGE (2018a), "Producao Agricola Municipal (PAM)," Instituto Brasileira de Geografia e Estatistica 2018. Available online: https://sidra.ibge.gov.br/pesquisa/pam/tabelas

IBGE (2018b), "Producao da Extracao Vegetal e da Silvicultura (PVES)," Instituto Brasileira de Geografia e Estatistica. Available online: https://sidra.ibge.gov.br/pesquisa/pevs/quadros/brasil/2018.

"Information Requested from the Department (for Paul Eaton) on FPC Program at College Park" (1966), Box 1 FPC Correspondence file August 5, 1965–February

1966, RG 22 Records concerning the Fish Protein Concentrate Program, 1959–1968, US National Archives and Records Administration.

"Ingredients" (n.d.), *Your Super*. Available online: https://yoursuper.com/pages/ingredients.

IPGRI. (2002), *Neglected No More*. International Plant Genetic Resources Institute and International Fund for Agricultural Development.

Ives, S. (2014), "Farming the South African 'Bush': Ecologies of Belonging and Exclusion in Rooibos Tea," *American Ethnologist*, 41 (4): 698–713.

Ives, S. (2017), *Steeped in Heritage: The Racial Politics of South African Rooibos Tea*, Durham, NC: Duke University Press.

Jackson, J. (2000), "Sophisticated Science: Judges Amazed by Students' Projects," *Sun Times*, April 6, 2000, Final ed. Proquest.

Jackson Lears, T. J. (1983), "From Salvation to Self-Realization: Advertising and the Therapeutic Roots of the Consumer Culture, 1880–1930," in R. Wightman Fox and T. J. Jackson Lears (eds), *The Culture of Consumption: Critical Essays in American History, 1880–1980*, New York: Pantheon Books.

Jacobsen, S. E. (2011), "The Situation for Quinoa and its Production in Southern Bolivia: From Economic Success to Environmental Disaster: Quinoa Production in Southern Bolivia," *Journal of Agronomy and Crop Science*, 197 (5): 390–9. https://doi.org/10.1111/j.1439-037X.2011.00475.x.

Jensen, S. (2008), *Gangs, Politics and Dignity in Cape Town*, Oxford: University of Chicago Press.

Jessop, B. (2006), "Spatial Fixes, Temporal Fixes, and Spatio-Temporal Fixes," in N. Castree and D. Gregory (eds), *David Harvey: A Critical Reader*, 142–66, Antipode Book Series, Malden, MA; Oxford: Blackwell Pub.

Johnston, J. (2008), "The Citizen-Consumer Hybrid: Ideological Tensions and the Case of Whole Foods Market," *Theory and Society*, 37 (3): 229–70.

Joly, P.-B. (2013), "On the Economics of Techno-scientific Promises," in M. Akrich, Y. Barthe, F. Muniesa and P. Mustar (eds), *Débordements : Mélanges Offerts à Michel Callon*, 203–21, Paris: Presses des Mines.

Joshi, D., S. Sood, R. Hosahatti, L. Kant, A. Pattanayak, A. Kumar, D. Yadav, and M. Stetter. (2018), "From Zero to Hero: The Past, Present and Future of Grain Amaranth Breeding," *Theoretical and Applied Genetics*, 131: 1807–23. https://doi.org/10.1007/s00122-018-3138-y.

Joy, D. (2007), "Regulatory Issues: FDA Considers Functional Foods," *Food Processing*, January. Available online: https://www.foodprocessing.com/articles/2007/009/.

Jürgens, G., H. F. Hoff, G. M. Chisolm III, and H. Esterbauer. (1987), "Modification of Human Serum Low Density Lipoprotein by Oxidation—Characterization and Pathophysiological Implications," *Chemistry and Physics of Lipids*, 45: 315–36.

Kaptchuk, T. J. and F. Miller. (2015), "Placebo Effects in Medicine," *The New England Journal of Medicine*, 373 (1): 8–9.

Katz, E. and E. Lazos. (2017), "The Rediscovery of Native 'Super-Foods' in Mexico," in B. Sebastia (ed.), *Eating Traditional Food: Politics, Identity and Practices*, 20–47, New York: Routledge.

Keahey, J. A. (2013), *Emerging Markets, Sustainable Methods: Political Economy Empowerment in South Africa's Rooibos Tea Sector*, PhD Thesis, Colorado State University.

Kerssen, T. M. (2015), "Food Sovereignty and the Quinoa Boom: Challenges to Sustainable Re-peasantisation in the Southern Altiplano of Bolivia," *Third World Quarterly*, 36 (3): 489–507. https://doi.org/10.1080/01436597.2015.1002992.

Kilpatrick, K. (2015), "The Aztec Superfood Fighting Mexican Obesity," *Al Jazeera America*. Available online: http://projects.aljazeera.com/2015/08/mexico-obesity/amaranth.html.

Kimura, A. H. (2013), *Hidden Hunger: Gender and the Politics of Smarter Foods*, Ithaca, NY: Cornell University Press.

Kimura, A. H., C. Biltekoff, J. Mudry, and J. Hayes-Conroy. (2014), "Nutrition as a Project," *Gastronomica*, 14 (3): 34–45.

Kiple, K. F. (ed.) (2000), *The Cambridge World History of Food*, Cambridge, UK: Cambridge University Press.

Kirshenblatt-Gimblett, B. and D. G. Fernandez. (2003), "Culture Ingested: On the Indigenization of Philippine Food," *Gastronomica*, 3 (1): 58–71.

Kline, W. (2001), *Building a Better Race: Gender, Sexuality, and Eugenics from the Turn of the Century to the Baby Boom*, Berkeley, CA: University of California Press.

Kloppenburg, J. (1988), *First the Seed: The Political Economy of Plant Biotechnology, 1492-2000*, New York: Cambridge University Press.

Knorr Cetina, K. (1999), *Epistemic Cultures: How the Sciences Make Knowledge*. Cambridge, MA: Harvard University Press.

Kopytoff, I. (1986), "The Cultural Biography of Things: Commoditization as Process," in A. Appadurai (ed.), *The Social Life of Things: Commodities in Cultural Perspective*, 64–92, Cambridge, UK: Cambridge University Press.

Kuli Kuli. (2019), *About Us*. Available online: https://www.kulikulifoods.com/about.

Lakoff, G. (1996), *Moral Politics*, Chicago, IL: University of Chicago Press.

Lakoff, G. and M. Johnson. (1980), *Metaphors We Live By*, Chicago, IL: University of Chicago Press.

Landecker, H. (2011), "Food as Exposure: Nutritional Epigenetics and the New Metabolism," *BioSocieties*, 6 (2): 167–94.

Landecker, H. (2013), "Postindustrial Metabolism: Fat Knowledge," *Public Culture*, 25 (3): 495–522. https://doi.org/10.1215/08992363-2144625.

Laskow, S. (2014), *A Distant Voyage, a Powerful Plant, and a Crowd-Backed Quest to Crack the Snack Market*. Available online: https://www.fastcompany.com/3029485/the-amazing-plant-powering-a-quest-to-crack-the-crowded-snack-market.

Latham, M. E. (2000), *Modernization as Ideology: American Social Science and "Nation Building" in the Kennedy Era*. Chapel Hill, NC: University of North Carolina Press.

Latour, B. (1993), *The Pasteurization of France*, Cambridge, MA: Harvard University Press.

Law, J. (2019), "Material Semiotics." Available online: www.heterogeneities.net/publications/Law2019MaterialSemiotics.pdf.

Le Page, M. (2018), "A New Kind of Superfood," *New Scientist*, 238 (3179): 28–32.

Leipold, S. and G. Winkel. (2016), "Divide and Conquer—Discursive Agency in the Politics of Illegal Logging in the United States," *Global Environmental Change*, 36: 35–45. https://doi.org/10.1016/j.gloenvcha.2015.11.006.

Levin, E. (1960), "Population Explosion and the Sea," Box 7 "FDA Fish Flour Background Information," RG 22 Records concerning the Fish Protein Concentrate Program, 1959–1968, National Archives and Records Administration, Maryland (US National Archives and Records Administration).

Levy, S. (2014), "Are Superfoods Really Good for You or Just Marketing Hype?" *Healthline*. Available online: https://www.healthline.com/health-news/superfoods-healthy-benefits-072214.

The Lexicon. (n.d.), *Rediscovered* [Website]. The Lexicon. Available online: https://www.thelexicon.org/rediscovered/.

Li, T. M. (2007), *The Will to Improve: Governmentality, Development, and the Practice of Politics*, Durham, NC: Duke University Press.

Li, X. and K. Siddique (eds) (2018), *Future Smart Food: Rediscovering Hidden Treasures of Neglected and Underutilized Species for Zero Hunger in Asia*, Bangkok: Food and Agriculture Organization.

Liboiron, M. (2013), "Plasticizers: A Twenty-First Century Miasma," in J. Gabrys, G. Hawkins and M. Michael (eds), *Accumulation: The Material Politics of Plastics*, 134–49, New York: Routledge.

Lizie, A. (2013), "Food and Communication," in K. Albala (ed.), *Routledge International Handbook of Food Studies*, 27–38, London and New York: Routledge.

Lombardo, P. A. (ed.) (2011), *A Century of Eugenics in America: From the Indiana Experiment to the Human Genome Era*, Bloomington, IN: Indiana University Press.

López-Garcia, R. (2008), "Amaranth: An Ancient Whole Grain from Mexico," *Cereal Foods World*, 53 (3): 155–6. https://doi.org/10.1094/CFW-53-3-0155.

Lost Crop of the Incas: Little-Known Plants of the Andes with Promise for Worldwide Cultivation. (1989), Washington, DC: National Research Council (NRC). http://www.nap.edu/openbook.php?record_id=1398&page=150.

Loyer, J. (2016a), "Communicating Superfoods: A Case Study of Maca Packaging," in M. McWilliams (ed.), *Food and Communication: Proceedings of the Oxford Symposium on Food and Cookery 2015*, 236–46, London: Prospect Books.

Loyer, J. (2016b), "Superfoods," in P. B. Thompson and D. M. Kaplan (eds), *Encyclopedia of Food and Agricultural Ethics*, 2nd ed., 1–7, Dordrecht: Springer Netherlands, https://doi.org/10.1007/978-94-007-6167-4_574-1.

Loyer, J. (2016c), *The Social Lives of Superfoods*, PhD Dissertation, University of Adelaide, School of Humanities.

Loyer, J. (2019), "Superfoods," in P. B. Thompson and D. M. Kaplan (eds), *Encyclopdia of Food and Agricultural Ethics*, 2269–75, Netherlands, Dordrecht: Springer.

Loyer, J. and C. Knight. (2018), "Selling the 'Inca Superfood': Nutritional Primitivism in Superfoods Books and Maca Marketing," *Food, Culture & Society*, 21 (4): 449–67. https://doi.org/10.1080/15528014.2018.1480645.

Lunn, J. (2006), "Superfoods," *Nutrition Bulletin*, 31 (3): 171–2. https://doi.org/10.1111/j.1467-3010.2006.00578.x.

Lybbert, T. J., N. Magnan, and A. Aboudrare. (2010), "Household and Local Forest Impacts of Morocco's Argan Oil Bonanza," *Environment and Development Economics*, 15 (4): 439–64. https://doi.org/10.1017/S1355770X10000136.

Macekura, S. J. (2015), *Of Limits and Growth: The Rise of Global Sustainable Development in the Twentieth Century*, New York: Cambridge University Press.

MacGregor, C., A. Petersen, and C. Parker. (2018), "Promoting a Healthier, Younger You: The Media Marketing of Anti-Ageing Superfood," *Journal of Consumer Culture*, 1–16.

Maghirang, R. (2006), *National Strategic Plan for Vegetables*. Proceedings of the Fourth Mindanao Vegetable Congress. Davao Convention and Trade Center, April 27–28.

MAGNA. (2018), "MAGNA Global Advertising Forecast: Winter Update," New York. Available online: https://magnaglobal.com/magna-advertising-forecasts-winter-2018-update/.

Maisto, M. (2011), *Rediscovering Amaranth, the Aztec Superfood*, Forbes. Available online at https://www.forbes.com/sites/michellemaisto/2011/12/05/meet-amaranth-quinoas-ancient-superfood-cousin/#7eb1a3b9ac9c

Manno, J. (2000), *Privileged Goods: Commoditization and its Implications for Environment and Society*, Boca Raton, FL: Lewis.

Manno, J. (2002), "Commoditization: Consumption Efficiency and an Economy of Care and Connection," in T. Princen, M. Maniates and K. Conca (eds), *Confronting Consumption*, 67–100, Cambridge: MIT Press.

Manno, J. (2010), "Commoditization and Oppression: A Systems Approach to Understanding the Economic Dynamics of Modes of Oppression," *Annals of the New York Academy of Science*, 1185: 164–78.

Mapes Sanchez, C. and F. B. Peña. (2016), "Los Quintoniles: Un recurso alimenticio milenario," *Arqueología Mexicana*, 23 (138): 34–9.

Markowitz, L. (2012), "Highland Haute Cuisine: The Transformation of Alpaca Meat," in E. Finnis (ed.), *Reimagining Marginalized Foods: Global Processes, Local Places*, 34–48, Tuscon: University of Arizona Press.

Marx, K. (1990 [1887]), *Capital*, vol. 1, London: Penguin.

Matejowsky, T. (2009), "Fast Food and Nutritional Perceptions in the Age of 'Globesity': Perspectives from the Provincial Philippines," *Food and Foodways*, 17: 29–49.

Matsumoto, N. (2017), "Why Mexican Chefs, Farmers and Activists Are Reviving the Ancient Grain Amaranth," *National Public Radio*, May 1. Available online: https://www.npr.org/sections/thesalt/2017/05/01/526033083/why-mexican-chefs-farmers-and-activists-are-reviving-the-ancient-grain-amaranth.

Mattill, H. A. and H. S. Olcott. (1937), "Method and Material for Retarding Oxidation and Rancidity in Food Substances," United States Patent Office 2098254, filed August 28, 1936, and issued November 9, 1937.

Mayer, E. (2009), *Ugly Stories of the Peruvian Agrarian Reform*, Durham, NC: Duke University Press.

McClung de Tapia, E. (2016), "El Amaranto desde el punto de vista arqueologico," *Arqueología Mexicana*, 23 (138): 22–5.

McDonell, E. (2015), "Miracle Foods: Quinoa, Curative Metaphors, and the Depoliticization of Global Hunger Politics," *Gastronomica: The Journal of Critical Food Studies*, 15: 70–85. https://doi.org/10.1525/gfc.2015.15.4.70.

McDonell, E. (2016), "Nutrition Politics in the Quinoa Boom: Connecting Consumer and Producer Nutrition in the Commercialization of Traditional Foods," *International Journal of Food and Nutritional Science*, 3 (6): 1–7.

McDonell, E. (2019a), "(Re)Producing 'Indian Food': Race, Value, and Development in Peru's Quinoa Boom-Bust," Dissertation, Indiana University.

McDonell, E. (2019b), "Creating the Culinary Frontier: A Critical Examination of Peruvian Chefs' Narratives of Lost/Discovered Foods," *Anthropology of Food*. https://doi.org/10.4000/aof.10183.

McKnight Foundation. (2020), "Project Overview," *Collaborative Crop Research Program*. Available online: https://www.ccrp.org/grants/quinoa-i/.

McLaren, D. (1966), "A Fresh Look at Protein-Calorie Malnutrition," *The Lancet*, 2 (7461): 485–8.

McLaren, D. S. (1974), "The Great Protein Fiasco," *The Lancet*, 304 (7872): 93–6.

McLeod-Kilmurray, H. (2012), "Commoditizing Non-human Animals and Their Consumers: Industrial Livestock Production, Animal Welfare, and Ecological Justice," *Bulletin of Science, Technology & Society*, 32 (1): 71–85.

Media Dynamics Inc. (2014), "American's Media Usage Trends and Ad Exposure: 1945–2014," Available online: https://www.mediadynamicsinc.com.

Meskell, L. (2012), *The Nature of Heritage*, Malden, MA: Wiley-Blackwell.

Mignolo, W. (2009), "Epistemic Disobedience, Independent Thought and Decolonial Freedom," *Theory Culture Society*, 26 (7–8): 159–81. https://doi.org/10.1177/0263276409349275.

Milner, C. (2015), "Science Loves This Superfood, So Why Aren't You Eating It?" Available online: www.theepochtimes.com.

Ministerio de Agricultura. (1973), Aspectos económicos en el cultivo de la quinua (provincios de Puno, Chucuito, Lampa, San Román, Dpto. de Puno), Zona Agraria XII (No. 20), Aspectos económicos, Ministerio de Agricultura, Oficina General de Estadística Lima.

Ministerio de Agricultura. (2014), "Quinua: Estadísticas de producción y exportación." 2014. Available online: https://www.inei.gob.pe/prensa/noticias/volumen-exportado-de-quinua-crecio-710-7455/

Mintel Press Team. (2016), "Super Growth for "Super" Foods: New Product Development Shoots Up 202% Globally over the Past Five Years," Mintel Global New Products Database.

Mintz, S. W. (1985), *Sweetness and Power: The Place of Sugar in Modern History*, New York: Penguin Books.

"A Miracle of the Fishes" (1962), *Life Magazine*, June 29: 33–4. Available online: https://books.google.com/books?id=_E0EAAAAMBAJ&printsec=frontcover.

Mol, A. (1999), "Ontological Politics. A Word and Some Questions," *The Sociological Review*, 47 (1_suppl): 74–89.

Molvar, K. (2018), "Is Your Superfood Mix Working Hard Enough for You?" *BLDG 25*, July 10. Available online: https://blog.freepeople.com/2018/07/is-your-superfood-mix-working-hard-enough-for-you.

Montefrio, M. J. F. (2012), "Privileged Biofuels, Marginalized Indigenous Peoples: The Co-Evolution of Biofuels Development in the Tropics," *Bulletin of Science, Technology and Society*, 32 (1): 41–55.

Montefrio, M. J. F. (2020), "Cosmopolitan Translations of Alternative Eating," *Agriculture and Human Values*, 37 (2): 479–94.

Montefrio, M. J. F., J. De Chavez, A. Contreras, and D. Erasga. (2020), "Hybridities and Awkward Constructions in Philippine Locavorism: Reframing Global-Local Dynamics through Assemblage Thinking," *Food, Culture & Society*, 23 (2): 117–36.

Moran, R. (2018), *Governing Bodies: American Politics and the Shaping of the Modern Physique*. Philadelphia, PA: University of Pennsylvania Press.

Morozov, E. (2013), "The Perils of Perfection," *The New York Times*. Available online: https://www.nytimes.com/2013/03/03/opinion/sunday/the-perils-of-perfection.html.

Mosse, D. (2013), "The Anthropology of International Development," *Annual Review of Anthropology*, 42 (1): 227–46. https://doi.org/10.1146/annurev-anthro-092412-155553.

Mourão, L. (1999), "Do açaí ao palmito: Uma história ecológica das permanencias, tensões e rupturas no estuário Amazônico," Tese de Doutorado, Nucleo de Altos Estudos Amazônicos, Universidade Federal do Pará, Belém.

Mudry, J. J. (2009), *Measured Meals: Nutrition in America*, Albany, NY: SUNY Press.

Mujica, A., S. E. Jacobsen, and J. Izquierdo. (2001a), "Resistencia a factores adversos de la quinua," in A. Mujica, S. E. Jacobsen, J. Izquierdo and J. P. Marathee (eds), *Quinua (Chenopodium Quinoa Willd.): Ancestral Cultivo Andino, Alimento Del Presente y Futuro*, 162–83, Santiago, Chile: FAO, UNA-Puno, CIP.

Mujica, A., S. E. Jacobsen, J. Izquierdo, and J. P. Marathee. (2001b), *Resultados de la Prueba Americana y Europea de la Quinua*, Puno: FAO, UNA & CIP.

Nader, R. (1965), *Unsafe at Any Speed: The Designed-In Dangers of the American Automobile*, New York: Grossman Publishers.

National Academy of Sciences (NAS). (1975), Underexploited Tropical Plants with Promising Economic Value, Report of an Ad Hoc Panel of the Advisory Committee on Technology Innovation, Board on Science and Technology for International Development, Commission on International Relations, National Academy of Science, Washington, DC.

National Institute of Health. (2017), "National Institute on Aging (NIA)," *The NIH Almanac* (blog), March 1, 2017. Available online: https://www.nih.gov/about-nih/what-we-do/nih-almanac/national-institute-aging-nia.

"Needs, Goals, and Objectives" (1967), Box 12 folder 1, RG 22 Records concerning the Fish Protein Concentrate Program, 1959–1968, US National Archives and Records Administration.

Nelder, C. (2013), "Positive energy," *Nature*, 498: 293–5. https://doi.org/10.1038/498293a.

Nelson, D. C. (1968), "Taxonomy and Origins of Chenopodium Quinoa and Chenopodium Nuttalliae," Ph.D. Dissertation. Indiana University Bloomington.

Nestle, M. (2013), *Food Politics: How the Food Industry Influences Nutrition and Health*, Revised and expanded tenth anniversary ed. Berkeley, Los Angeles, CA and London: University of California Press.

Nestle, M. (2018a), "Superfoods Are a Marketing Ploy," *The Atlantic*. Available online: https://www.theatlantic.com/health/archive/2018/10/superfoods-marketing-ploy/573583/.

Nestle, M. (2018b), *Unsavory Truth: How Food Companies Skew the Science of What We Eat*. New York: Basic Books.

Nichter, M. and J. J. Thompson. (2006), "For My Wellness, Not Just My Illness: North Americans' Use of Dietary Supplements," *Culture, Medicine and Psychiatry*, 30 (2): 175–222. https://doi.org/10.1007/s11013-006-9016-0.

Nkosi, N. (2018), "Drink It Up—The Health Benefits of Rooibos Tea Are Endless." Available online: https://www.destinyconnect.com/2018/08/08/6-amazing-benefits-of-rooibos-tea/.

Noble, M. (2018), "Bison Bars Were Supposed to Restore Native Communities and Grass-Based Ranches. Then Came Epic Provisions." *The Counter*. November 27. Available online: https://thecounter.org/tanka-bar-general-mills-epic-provisions-bison-bars/.

Nogrady, B. (2016), "Why There Is No Such Thing as a 'Superfood,'" *BBC Future*, February 24. Available online: http://www.bbc.com/future/story/20161124-why-there-is-no-such-thing-as-a-superfood.

Norgaard, K. M. (2011), *Living in Denial: Climate Change, Emotions, and Everyday Life*, Cambridge, MA: MIT Press.

Nugent, S. (1993), *Amazonian Caboclo Society: An Essay on Invisibility and Peasant Economy*, Oxford: BERG.

Nuritas. (2019), "Company Website." Available online: https://www.nuritas.com/.

Nyland, S. (2016), "8 Products You Didn't Know where Made from Quinoa," *OrganicCrops*. Available online: http://organiccrops.net/en/news/160321-8-products-you-didnt-know-were-made-from-Quinoa.php.

O'Hagan, L. A. (2019), "Celebrity Greens Kale and Seaweed were Long Considered Food of Last Resort," *The Conversation*. Available online: http://theconversation.com/celebrity-greens-kale-and-seaweed-were-long-considered-food-of-last-resort-124663.

Orlove, B. S. (2009), "The Past, the Present, and Some Possible Future of Adaptation," in N. Adger, I. Lorenzoni, and K. O'Brien (eds), *Adapting to Climate Change*, 131–63, Cambridge, MA: Cambridge University Press.

Ou, B., D. Huang, and M. Hampsch-Woodill. (2002), "Analysis of Antioxidant Activities of Common Vegetables Employing Oxygen Radical Absorbance Capacity (ORAC) and Ferric Reducing Antioxidant Power (FRAP) Assays: A Comparative Study," *Journal of Agricultural and Food Chemistry*, 50: 3122–8.

Padulosi, S. (2017), "Bring NUS Back to the Table!," *GREAT Insights*, 6 (4): 21–2.

Padulosi, S., N. Bergamini, and T. Lawrence (eds) (2011), Proceedings of the International Conference. Presented at the On-Farm Conservation of Neglected and Underutilized Species: Status, Trends and Novel Approaches to Cope with Climate Change, Rome: Biodiversity International, Frankfurt.

Padulosi, S., J. Thompson, and P. Rudebjer. (2013), *Fighting Poverty, Hunger and Malnutrition with Neglected and Underutilized Species (NUS): Needs, Challenges and the Way Forward*, Rome: Bioversity International.

Padulosi, S., K. Amaya, M. Jäger, E. Gotor, W. Rojas, and R. Valdivia. (2014), "A Holistic Approach to Enhance the use of Neglected and Underutilized Species: The Case of Andean Grains in Bolivia and Peru," *Sustainability*, 6: 1283–312. https://dx.doi.org/10.3390/su6031283.

Palanca, C. (2016), *The Gullet: Dispatches on Philippine Food*, Manila, Philippines: Anvil Publishing.

Parasecoli, F. (2017), *Knowing Where It Comes From: Labeling Traditional Foods to Compete in a Global Market*, Iowa City, IA: University of Iowa Press.

Paratore, M. (2013), *Kuli Kuli: The Next Superfood, and a Way to Support Women in West Africa*. Available online: https://ediblestartups.com/2013/12/04/kuli-kuli-the-next-superfood-and-a-way-to-support-women-in-west-africa/.

Pariser, E. R., M. B. Wallerstein, C. J. Corkery, and N. L. Brown. (1978), *Fish Protein Concentrate: Panacea for Protein Malnutrition?* Cambridge: MIT Press.

Parkin, K. J. (2007), *Food Is Love: Advertising and Gender Roles in Modern America*. Philadelphia, PA: University of Pennsylvania Press.

Paxson, H. (2010), "Locating Value in Artisan Cheese: Reverse-Engineering Terroir for New World Landscapes," *American Anthropologist*, 112 (3): 442–55.

Paynter, B. (2018), *Can This Superfood Company Help Stop Extremism?* Available online: https://www.fastcompany.com/90250850/can-this-superfood-company-help-stop-extremism.

Peña, D., L. Calvo, P. McFarland, and G. Valle. (eds) (2017), *Mexican-Origin Foods, Foodways, and Social Movements: Decolonial Perspectives*, Fayetteville, AR: University of Arkansas Press.

Penn, N. (2005), *The Forgotten Frontier: Colonist and Khoisan on the Cape's Northern Frontier in the 18th Century*, Cape Town: Double Storey.

"Peru Backs Cultivation of Quinoa as a Cereal (Special Cable to *The New York Times*)." (1937), *The New York Times* 8.

Petrini, C. (2007), *Slow Food Nation: Why Our Food Should Be Good, Clean, and Fair*. New York: Rizzoli Ex Libris.

Philpott, T. (2013), "Are Quinoa, Chia Seeds, and Other 'Superfoods' a Scam?" *Mother Jones*. Available online: https://www.motherjones.com/environment/2013/06/are-superfoods-quinoa-chia-goji-good-for-you/.

Pietta, P. G. (2000), "Flavonoids as Antioxidants," *Journal of Natural Products*, 63: 1035–42.

Pilcher, J. (2012), "Taco Bell, Maseca, and Slow Food: A Postmodern Apocalypse for Mexico's Peasant Cuisine?" in C. Counihan and P. Van Esterik (eds), *Food and Culture. A Reader*, 426–36, New York: Routledge.

Pilcher, J. M. (1998), *Que vivan los tamales! Food and the Making of Mexican Identity*, Albuquerque, NM: University of New Mexico Press.

Porter, T. M. (1996), *Trust in Numbers: The Pursuit of Objectivity in Science and Public Life*, Princeton, NJ: Princeton University Press.

Probyn, E. (2000), *Carnal Appetites: FoodSexIdentities*. New York and London: Routledge.

PROINPA/FAO. (2011), "Quinoa: An Ancient Crop to Contribute to World Food Security," FAO Regional Office for Latin America and the Caribbean, La Paz, Bolivia.

Provencher, V., J. Polivy, and C. Peter Herman. (2009), "Perceived Healthiness of Food. If It's Healthy, You Can Eat More!," *Appetite*, 52 (2): 340–4. https://doi.org/10.1016/j.appet.2008.11.005.

Pursell, C. W. (1969), "The Farm Chemurgic Council and the United States Department of Agriculture, 1935–1939," *Isis*, 60 (3): 307–17.

Quijano, A. (1999), "Colonialidad del poder, cultura, y conocimiento en América Latina," *Dispositio*, 24: 137–48.

Quinn, L. (2018), "The Great Kalespiracy," *The Hustle*. Available online: https://thehustle.co/kale-oberon-sinclair.

Rabinow, P. and N. Rose. (2006), "Biopower Today," *BioSocieties*, 1 (2): 195–217.

Rankin, K. N. (2001), "Governing Development: Neoliberalism, Microcredit, and Rational Economic Woman," *Economy and Society*, 30 (1): 18–37.

Rao, S. and C. Huggins (2017), "Sweet 'Success': Contesting Biofortification Strategies to Address Malnutrition in Tanzania," in J. Sumberg (ed.), *Agronomy for Development*, 104–20, London; New York: Earthscan, Routledge.

Rath, E. (2010), *Food and Fantasy in Early Modern Japan*, Berkeley: University of California Press.

Reardon, T., J. M. Codron, L. Busch, J. Bingen, and C. Harris. (1999), "Global Change in Agrifood Grades and Standards: Agribusiness Strategic Responses in Developing Countries," *The International Food and Agribusiness Management Review*, 2 (3–4): 421–35.

"Report of Subcommittee on Criteria Selection" (1967), Box 12 folder 1, RG 22 Records concerning the Fish Protein Concentrate Program, 1959–1968, US National Archives and Records Administration.

Rheinberger, H. J. (1997), *Toward a History of Epistemic Things: Synthesizing Proteins in the Test Tube*. Stanford, CA: Stanford University Press.

Rheinberger, H. J. (2005), "A Reply to David Bloor: 'Toward a Sociology of Epistemic Things,'" *Perspectives on Science*, 13: 3.

Risch, E. (1953), *The Quartermaster Crops: Organization, Supply, and Services, Vol. 1.* Washington, DC: Government Printing Office.

Robinson, R. G. (1986), *Amaranth, Quinoa, Ragi, Tef, and Niger : Tiny Seeds of Ancient History and Modern Interest*, Minneapolis: Agricultural Experiment Station, University of Minnesota.

Rogez, H. (2000), *Açaí: Preparo, composição e melhoramento da conservação*, Belem: Editora da Universidade Federal do Pará.

Rojas-Rivas, E., A. Espinoza-Ortega, H. Thomé-Ortíz, S. S. Moctezuma-Pérez, and F. Cuffia. (2019), "Understanding Consumers' Perception and Consumption Motives towards Amaranth in Mexico Using the Pierre Bourdieu's Theoretical Concept of Habitus," *Appetite*, 139: 180–8. https://doi.org/10.1016/j.appet.2019.04.021.

Rose, N. (1992), "Governing the Enterprising Self," in P. Heelas and P. Morris (eds), *The Values of the Enterprise Culture: The Moral Debate*, 150–68, London; New York: Routledge.

Rose, N. (2001), "The Politics of Life Itself," *Theory, Culture & Society*, 18 (6): 1.

Rosner, L. (ed.) (2004), *The Technological Fix: How People Use Technology to Create and Solve Problems*, New York: Routledge.

Rudebjer, P., G. Meldrum, S. Padulosi, R. Hall, and E. Hermanowicz. (2014), *Realizing the Promise of Neglected and Underutilized Species*. Policy Brief. Bioversity International.

Ruiz, K., S. Biondi, R. Oses, I. Acuña-Rodríguez, F. Antognoni et al. (2014), "Quinoa Biodiversity and Sustainability for Food Security under Climate Change. A Review. Agronomy for Sustainable Development," *Springer Verlag/EDP Sciences/INRA*, 34 (2): 349–59.

Russell, P. (2015), *The Essential History of Mexico: From Pre-Conquest to Present*, London; New York: Routledge.

Ruxin, J. (2000), "The United Nations Protein Advisory Group," in D. F. Smith and J. Phillips (eds), *Food, Science, Policy and Regulation in the Twentieth Century: International and Comparative Perspectives*, 151–66, New York: Routledge.

Saillant, F., M. È. Drouin, and N. Gordon. (2012), "Formes, contenus et usages du témoignage dans les ONG d'aide internationale: La vérité à l'épreuve du marketing," *Alterstice—Revue Internationale de la Recherche Interculturelle*, 1 (2): 35–46.

Saker, V. A. (1990), "Benevolent Monopoly: The Legal Transformation of Agricultural Cooperation, 1890-1943," PhD Dissertation, University of California Berkeley.

Salmon, C. (2010), *Storytelling: Bewitching the Modern Mind*, London; New York: Verso.

Sandra Kruger and Associates. (2009), *Rooibos Socio-Economic Study*, public version, Pniel, SA: Ministry of Agriculture, Nature, and Food Quality.

Santos, B. D. S. (2011), "Épistémologies du Sud," *Etudes Rurales*, 187: 21–49.

"A Satisfactory Process for the Manufacture of Fish Protein Concentrate (Fish Flour)" (1961), Box 7 "FDA Fish Flour Background Information," RG 22 Records concerning the Fish Protein Concentrate Program, 1959–1968, US National Archives and Records Administration.

Scharff, C. (2016), "The Psychic Life of Neoliberalism: Mapping the Contours of Entrepreneurial Subjectivity," *Theory, Culture & Society*, 33 (6): 107–22. https://doi.org/10.1177/0263276415590164.

Schiemer, C., A. M. S. Halloran, K. Jespersen, and P. Kaukua (2018), "Marketing Insects: Superfood or Solution-Food?" in A. Halloran, R. Flore, P. Vantomme, and N. Roos (eds), *Edible Insects in Sustainable Food Systems*, 213–36, Cham: Springer.

Schmink, M. (2011), "Forest Citizens: Changing Life Conditions and Social Identities in the Land of the Rubber Tappers," *Latin American Research Review*, 46: 141–58.

Schneider, M. and P. McMichael. (2011), "Food Security Politics and the Millennium Development Goals," *Third World Quarterly*, 32 (1): 119–39. https://doi.org/10.1080/01436597.2011.543818.

Schoenberger, E. (2004), "The Spatial Fix Revisited," *Antipode*, 36 (3): 427–33. https://doi.org/10.1111/j.1467-8330.2004.00422.x.

Schroeder, R. (1993), "Shady Practice—Gender and the Political Ecology of Resource Stabilization in Gambian Garden Orchards," *Economic Geography*, 69 (4): 349–65.

Scrimshaw, N. and J. Gordon (eds) (1968), *Malnutrition, Learning, and Behavior*, Cambridge: MIT Press.

Scrinis, G. (2008), "On the Ideology of Nutritionism," *Gastronomica*, 8 (1): 39–48. https://doi.org/10.1525/gfc.2008.8.1.39.

Scrinis, G. (2013), *Nutritionism: The Science and Politics of Dietary Advice*, New York: Columbia University Press.

Sen, A. (1981), *Poverty and Famines: An Essay on Entitlement and Deprivation*, New York: Oxford University Press.

Sexton, A., T. Garnett, and J. Lorimer. (2019), "Framing the Future of Food: The Contested Promises of Alternative Proteins," *Environment and Planning E: Nature and Space*, 2 (1): 47–72. https://doi.org/10.1177/2514848619827009.

Shamsian, J. (2016), "A Food Critic Who Helped Make Kale Popular Now Thinks it is Totally Overrated," *Insider*. Available online: https://www.insider.com/food-critic-mimi-sheraton-kale-popular-overrated-2016-6.

Shapin, S. (2011), *Changing Tastes: How Foods Tasted in the Early Modern Period and How They Taste Now*, The Hans Rausing Lecture, Salvia Småskrifter 14, Uppsala.

Sheraton, M. (1976), "For Cold Nights, Kale Dishes Like Those the Norsemen Eat," *The New York Times*, January 8. Available online: https://www.nytimes.com/1976/01/28/archives/for-cold-nights-kale-dishes-like-those-the-norsemen-eat.html.

Shiva, V. (2007), "Bioprospecting as Sophisticated Biopiracy," *Signs: Journal of Women in Culture and Society*, 32 (2): 307–13. https://doi.org/10.1086/508502.

Shotwell, A. (2016), *Against Purity: Living Ethically in Compromised Times*, Minneapolis, MN: University of Minnesota Press.

Sifferlin, A. (2016), "The 50 Healthiest Foods of All Time (with Recipes)," *Time Magazine*. Available online: http://time.com/3724505/healthy-recipes-healthiest-foods/.

Sikka, T. (2016/2017), "Contemporary Superfood Cults: Nutritionism, Neoliberalism, and Gender," in K. Cargill (ed.), *Food Cults: How Fads, Dogma, and Doctrine Influence Diet*, 87–108, Lanham, MA: Rowman and Littlefield.

Sikka, T. (2019), "The Contradictions of a Superfood Consumerism in a Postfeminist, Neoliberal World," *Food, Culture, and Society*, 22 (3): 354–75. https://doi.org/10.1080 /15528014.2019.1580534.

Siqueira, A. D. and E. S. Brondizio. (2012), "Açaí, *Euterpe oleracea* mart," in J. P. Poulain (ed.), *Dictionnaire des cultures alimentaires*, 391–400, Paris: Presses Universitaires de France (PUF), 1488 p.

Sismondo, S. and J. A. Greene. (2015), *The Pharmaceutical Studies Reader*, Malden, MA: John Wiley & Sons.

Skrabanek, P. (1994), *The Death of Humane Medicine and the Rise of Coercive Healthism*, London, UK: Social Affairs Unit.

Smith, N. (2008), *Uneven Development: Nature, Capital, and the Production of Space*, Athens, GA: University of Georgia Press.

Smith-Howard, K. (2013), *Pure and Modern Milk: An Environmental History since 1900*, New York: Oxford University Press.

Sonnad, N. (2017), "All the 'Wellness' Products Americans Love to Buy Are Sold on Both Infowars and Goop." *Quartz*. Available online: https://qz.com/1010684/all-the-wellness-products-american-love-to-buy-are-sold-on-both-infowars-and-goop/.

South African Food Review. (2018), "How South Africans Like Their Rooibos," Available online: https://www.foodreview.co.za/how-south-africans-drink-rooibos/.

South African Rooibos Council. (2019), "Rooibos Research Gets Multi-Million Rand Boost," Available online: https://sarooibos.co.za/rooibos-research-gets-multi-million-rand-boost/.

Spackman, C. (2014), "Functional Foods," in P. B. Thompson and D. M. Kaplan (eds), *Encyclopedia of Food and Agricultural Ethics*, Dordrecht: Springer. https://doi.org/10.1007/978-94-007-0929-4.

Star, S. L. (1985), "Scientific Work and Uncertainty," *Social Studies of Science*, 15: 391–427.

Star, S. L. (2010), "This Is Not a Boundary Object," *Science, Technology and Human Values*, 35: 601–17.

Starr, P. (1982), *The Social Transformation of American Medicine*, New York: Basic Books.

Statistics South Africa. (2017), "Mid-Year Population Estimates." Available online: https://www.statssa.gov.za/publications/P0302/P03022017.pdf.

Stecker, M. J. (2016), "Awash in a Sea of Confusion: Benefit Corporations, Social Enterprise, and the Fear of 'Greenwashing'," *Journal of Economic Issues*, 50 (2): 373–81. https://doi.org/10.1080/00213624.2016.1176481.

Steinberg, D. (1995), "Clinical Trials of Antioxidants in Atherosclerosis: Are We Doing the Right Thing?" *The Lancet*, 346 (8966): 36–8.

Steinberg, D. (2009), "The LDL Modification Hypothesis of Atherogenesis: An Update," *Journal of Lipid Research*, 50 (Suppl.): S376–81.

Sterling-Rice Group. (2018), "You and Almonds VS." Available online: https://www.srg.com/case-studies/abc-vs.php.

Stern, A. (2016), *Eugenic Nation: Faults and Frontiers of Better Breeding in Modern America*, Berkeley, CA: University of California Press.

Stoll, S. (1998), *The Fruits of Natural Advantage: Making the Industrial Countryside in California*. Berkeley, CA: University of California Press.

"Superfoods Market by Product and Geography—Forecast and Analysis 2020–2024" 2020. Technavio.

"Superfoods or Superhype?" (2018), *The Nutrition Source*, Harvard T.H. Chan School of Public Health. Available online: https://www.hsph.harvard.edu/nutritionsource/superfoods/.

Swinbanks, D. and J. O'Brien. (1993), "Japan Explores the Boundary between Food and Medicine," *Nature*, 364: 180.

Tapia, M. E. (2000), *Cultivos andinos subexplotados y su aporte a la alimentación*, 2nd ed., Santiago, Chile: Oficina Regional de la FAO para América Latina y el Caribe.

Technavio. (2018), "Global Superfoods Market 2018–2022," Market Research. London, UK. Available online: https://www.technavio.com/report/global-super-foods-market-analysis-share-2018.

Technavio. (2020), "Superfoods Market by Product and Geography—Forecast and Analysis 2020–2024." London, UK.

Thier, D. (2010), "The Story of a Cursed Crop," *The Atlantic*. Available online: https://www.theatlantic.com/health/archive/2010/01/quinoa-the-story-of-a-cursed-crop/33638/

Torres, H. A. (1980). *Escarificadora de quinua diseno y construccion*. IICA Biblioteca Venezuela.

Tsai, L. (2013), *Kuli Kuli: Oakland Startup Touts West African "Superfood."* Available online: https://www.eastbayexpress.com/WhatTheFork/archives/2013/12/10/kuli-kuli-oakland-startup-touts-west-african-superfood.

Tsing, A. (2015), *The Mushroom at the End of the World: On the Possibility of Life in Capitalist Ruins*. Princeton, NJ: Princeton University Press.

Tsing, A. L. (2013), "Sorting Out Commodities: How Capitalist Value is Made through Gifts," *HAU: Journal of Ethnographic Theory*, 3 (1): 21–43.

Tucker, T. C. (1920), "The Future of the California Almond," Blue Diamond Brand, UC Davis Special Collections.

Türken, S., H. E. Nafstad, R. M. Blakar, and K. Roen. (2016), "Making Sense of Neoliberal Subjectivity: A Discourse Analysis of Media Language on Self-Development," *Globalizations*, 13 (1): 32–46. https://doi.org/10.1080/14747731.2015.1033247.

Turner, B. (2014), "Neoliberal Politics of Resource Extraction: Moroccan Argan Oil," *Forum for Development Studies*, 41 (2): 207–32. https://doi.org/10.1080/08039410.2014.901239.

Turner, M. (2015), "Experts say Superfoods may be a Super Scam," *The Daily Universe*. Available online: https://universe.byu.edu/2015/09/22/experts-say-superfoods-may-be-a-super-scam1/.

UC Davis. (2018), "What Makes Superfood So Super?" Available online: https://www.ucdavis.edu/food/what-makes-superfood-so-super.

United Nations, Department of Economic and Social Affairs. (1971), *Strategy Statement on Action to Avert the Protein Crisis in the Developing Countries*, New York: United Nations.

United States Department of Agriculture (USDA). (2014), "2012 Census of Agriculture." Available online: https://www.nass.usda.gov/Publications/AgCensus/2012/Full_Report/Volume_1,_Chapter_1_US/usv1.pdf.

United States Department of Agriculture (USDA). (2019), "2017 Census of Agriculture." Available online: https://www.nass.usda.gov/Publications/AgCensus/2017/Full_Report/Volume_1,_Chapter_1_US/usv1.pdf.

United States Department of Agriculture (2018), "Fruit and Tree Nut Yearbook Tables," Economic Research Report. United States Department of Agriculture, Economic Research Service. Available online: https://www.ers.usda.gov/data-products/fruit-and-tree-nut-data/fruit-and-tree-nut-yearbook-tables/.

"U.S. State Department Threatens to Withdraw Aid from Peru and Ecuador in Connection with Fisheries Controversy" (1967), *Andean Air Mail & Peruvian Times*, March 3, Box 2 folder 1, RG 22 Records concerning the Fish Protein Concentrate Program, 1959–1968, US National Archives and Records Administration.

Van der Ploeg, J. D. (2012), *The New Peasantries: Struggles for Autonomy and Sustainability in an Era of Empire and Globalization*. London, Stirling, VA: Earthscan.

Van Esterik, P. (2006), "From Hunger Foods to Heritage Foods: Challenges to Food Localization in LAO PDR," in R. Wilk (ed.), *Fast Food/Slow Food: The Cultural Economy of the Global Food System*, 83–96, Lanham, MD: Altamira Press.

Vargas Guadarrama, L. alberto, and M. del Valle Berrocal. (2016), "El nuevo reventón del amaranto," *Arqueologia Mexicana*, 23 (138): 59–63.

Vega-Gálvez, A., M. Miranda, J. Vergara, E. Uribe, L. Puente, and E. A. Martínez. (2010), "Nutrition Facts and Functional Potential of Quinoa (Chenopodium quinoa willd.), an Ancient Andean Grain: A Review," *Journal of the Science of Food and Agriculture*, 90: 2541–7. https://doi.org/10.1002/jsfa.4158.

Veit, H. Z. (2015), *Modern Food, Moral Food: Self-Control, Science and the Rise of Modern American Eating in the Early Twentieth Century*. Chapel Hill, NC: University of North Carolina Press.

Velasco Lozano, A. M. (2016), "Los cuerpos divinos: El amaranto: comida ritual y cotidiana," *Arqueologia Mexicana*, 23 (138): 26–33.

Velasco Lozano, A. M. (2017), "El amaranto, un recurso alimenticio de larga duración. Patrimonio Cultural Intangible de la Ciudad de Mexico," *Boletin Colegio de Etnologos y Antropologos Sociales*. 65–73.

Venskutonis, P. and P. Kraujalis. (2013), "Nutritional Components of Amaranth Seeds and Vegetables: A Review on Composition, Properties, and Uses," *Comprehensive Reviews in Food Science and Food Safety*, 12: 381–412. https://doi.org/10.1111/1541-4337.12021.

Villela Flores, S. (2016), "El huauhtli sagrado: los tamales tzoalli entre los Nahuas de Guerrero," *Arqueología Mexicana*, 23 (138): 46–53.

Viñas, E. T. (1953), *Relación entre el contenido de aminoácidos esenciales y el valor nutritivo de la proteina de la quinua. Actas Del Cuarto Congreso Peruano*, Lima, Perú: de Quimica.

Vollenhoven, S. (Producer) (2018), *Rooibos Restitution* [Motion Picture]. South Africa: Heinrich Böll Foundation.

Waite, M. (2018), *Kuli Kuli: A Superstar of Superfoods*. Available online: https://www.greenbiz.com/article/kuli-kuli-superstar-superfoods.

Walker, M., S. M. Roberts, J. P. Jones et al. (2008), "Neoliberal Development through Technical Assistance: Constructing Communities of Entrepreneurial Subjects in Oaxaca, Mexico," *Geoforum*, 39 (1): 527–42. https://doi.org/10.1016/j.geoforum.2007.10.009.

Walvin, J. (1997), *Fruits of Empire*, New York: New York University Press.

Wang, H., G. Cao, and R. L. Prior (1997), "Oxygen Radical Absorbing Capacity of Anthocyanins," *Journal of Agricultural and Food Chemistry*, 45: 304–9.

Wang, H., G. Cao, and R. L. Prior. (1996), "Total Antioxidant Capacity of Fruits," *Journal of Agricultural and Food Chemistry*, 44: 701–5.

Wayland, C. (2003), "Contextualizing the Politics of Knowledge: Physicians' Attitudes toward Medicinal Plants," *Medical Anthropology Quarterly*, 17: 483–500.

Weber, E. J. (1978), "A New Start for an Ancient Crop," *International Development Research Centre (IDRC) Reports*, 7: 2–4.

Weinstein, S. and S. Moegenburg. (2004), "Açaí Palm Management in the Amazon Estuary: Course for Conservation or Passage to Plantations?" *Conservation & Society*, 2 (2): 315–46.

Weis, T. (2007), *The Global Food Economy: The Battle for the Future of Farming*, London: Zed Books.

Weismantel, M. J. (2000), "The Children Cry for Bread: Hegemony and the Transformation of Consumption," in A. H. Goodman, D. L. Dufour, and G. H. Pelto (eds), *Nutritional Anthropology*, 136–44, Mountain View, CA: Mayfield.

West, P. (2012), *From Modern Production to Imagined Primitive: The Social World of Coffee from Papua New Guinea*. Durham, NC: Duke University Press.

White, P. L., E. Alvistur, C. Dias, E. Viñas, H. S. White, and C. Collazos. (1955), "Nutritive Values of Crops, Nutrient Content and Protein Quality of Quinua and Cañihua, Edible Seed Products of the Andes Mountains," *Journal of Agricultural and Food Chemistry*, 3: 531–4. https://doi.org/10.1021/jf60052a009.

Wild Blueberry Association of North America. (2008), "Blueberry Juice Tops the ORAC Antioxidant Chart," May 5, 2008. Available online: https://www.wildblueberries.com/?pressreleases=blueberry-juice-tops-the-orac-antioxidant-chart.

Wilk, R. (2006), *Home Cooking the Global Village: Caribbean Food from Buccaneers to Ecotourists*, Oxford and New York: Berg.

Wilk, R. (2008), "A Taste of Home: The Cultural and Economic Significance of European Food Exports to the Colonies," in A. Nuetzenadel and F. Trentmann (eds), *Food and Globalization: Consumption, Markets and Politics in the Modern World*, 93–109, Oxford: Berg.

Wilk, R. (2012), "Water Magic," in H. P. Hahn, K. Cless, and J. Soentgen (eds), *People at the Well: Kinds, Usages and Meanings of Water in a Global Perspective*, 126–44, Frankfurt: Campus Verlag.

Wilmsen, E. (1989), *Land Filled with Flies: A Political Economy of the Kalahari*, Chicago, IL: University of Chicago Press.

Wilson, K. (2015), "A Bitter Victory," *FSR Magazine*. Available online: https://www. foodnewsfeed.com/fsr/bitter-victory.

Winders, W. (2009), *The Politics of Food Supply: U.S. Agricultural Policy in the World Economy*, New Haven, CT: Yale University Press. Available online: http://public. eblib.com/choice/publicfullrecord.aspx?p=3420615.

Wolfe, D. (2009), *Superfoods: The Food and Medicine of the Future*, Berkeley, CA: North Atlantic Books.

Wynberg, R. (2017), "Making Sense of Access and Benefit Sharing in the Rooibos Industry: Towards a Holistic, Just and Sustainable Framing," *South African Journal of Botany*, 110: 39–51.

Wynberg, R. (2019), "San and Khoi Claim Benefits from Rooibos," *Mail and Guardian*. Available online: https://mg.co.za/article/2019-11-01-00-san-and-khoi-claim-benefits-from-rooibos.

Wynberg, R., D. Schroeder, and R. Chennells (eds) (2009), *Indigenous Peoples, Consent and Benefit-Sharing: Lessons from the San-Hoodia Case*, London and New York: Springer.

Wynberg, R., S. Laird, J. Van Niekerk, and W. Kozanayi. (2015), "Formalization of the Natural Product Trade in Southern Africa: Unintended Consequences and Policy Blurring in Biotrade and Bioprospecting," *Society & Natural Resources*, 28 (5): 559–74. https://doi.org/10.1080/08941920.2015.1014604.

Yates-Doerr, E. (2015), "The Opacity of Reduction: Nutritional Black-Boxing and the Meanings of Nourishment," *Food, Culture, and Society*, 15 (2): 293–313. https://doi. org/10.2752/175174412X13233545145381.

"The Year's Opportunity" (1920), *American Nut Journal*, 12 (1): 8.

Zimmerman, C. C. (1932), "Ernst Engel's Law of Expenditures for Food," *The Quarterly Journal of Economics*, 47 (1): 78. https://doi.org/10.2307/1885186.

Zins, M. (2016), "Five 'Super' Crops That Can Change the World," *IFAD Social Reporting Blog*, May 20, 2016.

Index

agency 170, 176
    institutional 3, 169
agricultural monocultures 100
agrobiodiversity 180, 184
agroforestry 152–7
American consumer 17, 79–81, 84
amino acids 80, 97, 173, 179
anti-aging properties 32, 39, 71, 119, 159
antioxidants 39–46, 57–75, 122, 157, 159
Appadurai, Arjun 39, 136–7, 147
Aztec 10, 174, 176

benefit sharing 40, 51–3
biodiversity 152, 166, 171
biofortification 174
biomedicalization 60
biopolitics 131
bioprospecting 11–12, 45, 47, 61, 88, 100
biotechnology 173
boom-bust cycles 8–9, 24
boundary object 3, 9, 96, 115–17, 128–9,
    158

cancer prevention 37, 46, 141, 180
charismatic nutrients 7, 89, 97, 124, 129,
    131
cholesterol 29, 65, 180
climate change benefits 102, 111–13, 180
climate smart crops 80, 180
cognitive performance 32, 120–2
colonialism 43, 49, 125, 139, 169, 171, 175,
    185
colorful foods 57, 68, 73–4, 123
comida de indios 96–7, 170
commodity 19–20, 135–8, 140–8, 153, 165
    fetish 39, 43, 50, 115, 136, 158, 175, 185
    potentials 137–8, 140–6
contaminated food 8, 122, 130, 163
contract growers 142
counter cuisine 131
credence qualities 137, 141–2, 147
culinary revalorization 170

decolonization 183, 185
depoliticization of malnutrition 7, 184
deregulation 5
dietary supplement 5, 63–4, 89
discourse 20–2, 39, 96–103
    analysis 170–5
drug foods 1, 5–6

economic benefits for women 178–9
ethical capitalism 123, 130, 161
extractionist logic 58–9, 73, 75, 175
extractivism 154–8

farm-to-table 135, 139–40, 144
farmer's markets 140
fashion foods 157, 160
fast food 9, 23, 139, 171
Foucault, Michel 20
functional foods 5, 21–2, 58, 61–4, 73, 75,
    120, 130

General Mills 91
genetic modification 44
    non-GMO 119, 122
geographic indications 45
global hunger 102, 126, 180
government aid 19, 152, 165
governmental bodies
    Peru
        Ministry of Agriculture and
            Alimentation 108
        Ministry of Exterior Commerce 1
    South Africa
        Department of Environmental
            Affairs 47, 50
        National Khoisan Council 47, 50
        South African San Council 47, 50
    United States
        Bureau of Commercial Fisheries
            127–8
        Department of Agriculture 25–7,
            60, 69, 98, 127

Department of Interior 119
FDA 29, 62–4
Foreign Market Development
  Program 27
NASA 176, 180
National Academy of Sciences 63,
  98, 176
National Food and Nutrient
  Analysis Program 69
National Institute on Aging 64
National Research Council 98,
  107
USAID 83, 86, 128
green revolution 98–9, 183
greenwashing 90

health benefits (individual) 60, 120
  breathing 41
  depression 180
  diabetes 141
  gut function 32, 72
  hair 41
  immune system 72, 122
  mood 121
  Parkinson's disease 37
  probiotic 6
  sexual 37, 72
  sleep 37
  strength 119
health food 109, 172
healthism 88–9
heart disease 29, 35, 141, 180
heritage 12, 38, 51, 171–2, 180
home growers 87, 135, 138, 144–7

Inca 102, 105, 174
Indigeneity 9, 40, 122, 171
  authenticity 49, 51
  foodways 69–70, 158, 171
  identity 149, 157
indigenization 139, 145
industrialization 136, 160–2, 171
industry conventions 10, 79
intellectual property 12, 184
intercropping 154, 156
international development 4, 95–117,
  152
  development potential 8, 96, 101–2,
    116

Kellogg 84–5, 91, 176–7, 183
Khoisan 46–52
knowledge
  Indigenous 162
  intangible 46, 48
  intergenerational 21
  local 88, 156
  scientific 44, 60–1
    and state authority 22
  traditional 12, 40, 46–53, 122, 156, 180

land rights 47–8, 155–6
Latour, Bruno 3, 67

magical qualities 3, 157, 159, 161
malnutrition 102, 105–7, 127, 178
marketing 23, 35
  celebrities 135, 138, 161, 180
  and entrepreneurs 41–2, 110–11
  and gender 23, 27, 34
  influencers 138
  and nostalgia 34
  self-care 42
  social media 141
  and "tradition" 119, 122
Marx, Karl 20, 38, 50
materiality 43, 66–9, 138, 147
Maya 174–5
miracle crops 80, 82, 95–117, 149, 174
miracle foods 7, 80, 149, 159, 174, 182
modernization theory 126, 171

narratives 153, 159, 169–85
  discovery narratives 170, 173, 178
  female empowerment 83, 92
  forgotten foods narratives 177–9
  future smart food 182
  neglected crops 182
  panacea narratives 22, 175, 180
  promissory narratives 179–81
  slow food 182
national identity 38, 139
neocolonialism 166, 183
Nestlé 23, 45, 54
NGOs 176
  American Heart Association 29, 41
  Arab Bank for Economic Development
    in Africa 113
  Biodiversity International 101, 112, 182

Clinton Foundation 80, 84
Inter-American Development Bank
    101
Inter-American Institute for
    Cooperation on Agriculture 108
International Centre for Underutilized
    Crops 101
McKnight Foundation 104
*Promocion e Investigacion de Productos
    Andinos* 104
World Health Organization 124, 180
nutritional primitivism 11, 122–3, 175,
    178
nutritional reductionism 58, 68
nutritional science 2, 53, 61
nutritionism 22, 61, 88–90, 123

ORAC 57–8, 66–70, 73–5

packaging 13, 70, 79, 119
poverty 102, 107–11, 180
processed food 4, 8, 23
production of superfoods 34, 158, 162–5
    expansion 158–62
    impact of consumer markets on
        farmers 26, 28, 96, 142–5
    protein gap 97, 125–6, 129–30

race 123, 125, 156, 169
    ambiguity 40, 46–7
    the other 11–12

seasonality 24–5
semiotics 18–20, 152, 157–62
skin health 37, 41, 121–2
small-scale producers 135, 152–3, 156,
    165–6
social class identities 169
sociology of expectations 170
solutionism 7, 79–93, 103
spatial fix 18–20, 33–6
structuralism 3
style sandwich 138
super-commodity 54
superfoods
    decline 10, 13, 148
    definition of 41, 89, 123, 130–1, 173
    ecological indigeneity 38–9
    failed 10

local 148
market size 1, 17
military usage 97
overproduction 28, 34–6
ownership 45
regulation 22, 47, 58–63
seeds 142–3, 145, 184
as snacks 32, 90, 158
as soft diplomacy 127
supply chain logistics 147, 152
value aggregation 152–3, 157–64
sustainability 152, 157–8

taste 8, 60, 73, 83
trade organizations
    Almond Board of California 18
    Almond Control Board (Blue
        Diamond Growers) 26–33
    American Dietetic Association 62
    California Almond Growers Exchange
        24–6, 28
    South African Rooibos Council
        51
    Wild Blueberry Association 69–70
transformation of superfoods 11, 70, 74–5,
    143, 158
    alcoholic 42, 161
    beverages 84, 158
    concentrates 158
    cosmetics 158, 161
    dehydration 124, 143
    desserts 158
    energy bars 143
    frying 172
    and gender 159
    infusion 37
    juicing 142, 145
    medication 161
    powders 42, 84, 90, 119–32, 143,
        158
    roasting/grinding 161
    skincare 42

underfoods 8
understanding of place 39–40, 46
United Nations 96
    Food and Agriculture Organization
        101–2, 106, 112, 116, 124,
        182

International Fund for Agricultural
    Development 177
International Year of Quinoa 96, 106,
    113–16
Protein Advisory Group 125
UNESCO 171
UNICEF 108
urban farming 144

vegetarianism 131, 140
venture capital 79–88, 92, 121
    disruption 7, 79, 81

weight loss 35, 119, 121–2, 142,
    178
whole foods 5, 21, 28, 69

www.ingramcontent.com/pod-product-compliance
Lightning Source LLC
Chambersburg PA
CBHW050431280326
41932CB00013BA/2066